Weight-Loss Surgery with the Adjustable Gastric Band

ROBERT W. SEWELL, M.D., F.A.C.S., is an award-winning laparoscopic surgeon. His articles have been published in numerous medical journals and professional books, and he is a frequent speaker at medical conferences. Dr. Sewell has taught laparoscopic techniques all over the world, and he has over 300 AGB patients. He lives outside Dallas, Texas.

LINDA ROHRBOUGH is a best-selling author and patient of Dr. Sewell's. Rohrbough received a *LAP-BAND®* in early 2004 and has subsequently lost 136 pounds. She lives outside Dallas, Texas.

Weight-Loss Surgery with the Adjustable Gastric Band

Everything You Need to Know
Before and After Surgery
to Lose Weight Successfully

Robert W. Sewell, M.D., F.A.C.S.

Linda Rohrbough

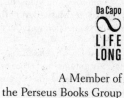

Da Capo
LIFE
LONG

A Member of
the Perseus Books Group

Designed by Jeff Williams

Cataloging-in-Publication data for this book is available from the Library of Congress.

First Da Capo Press edition 2008
ISBN 978-1-60094-002-6

Published by Da Capo Press
A Member of the Perseus Books Group
www.dacapopress.com

Da Capo Press books are available at special discounts for bulk purchases in the United States by corporations, institutions, and other organizations. For more information, please contact the Special Markets Department at the Perseus Books Group, 2300 Chestnut Street, Suite 200, Philadelphia, PA 19103, or call (800) 255-1514, or e-mail special.markets@perseusbooks.com.

10 9 8 7 6 5 4 3 2 1

Contents

Preface

Dear Reader,

Any time you pick up a book that has anything to do with healthcare, there will invariably be some type of disclaimer. It seems that such things are necessary, even though it should be obvious to everyone that the material in any book is by its very nature meant for the general public, not as a specific recommendation for any individual. The following paragraph is our disclaimer.

The material contained in this book is intended solely for informational purposes. It is not a replacement for an individual consultation with your personal physician. It is not the intention here either to make a diagnosis or to recommend a specific treatment for any medical or psychological condition. In the event that any information contained in this book seems to conflict with the opinions or recommendations of your personal physician, you should rely on his or her judgment, since that is based on a personal knowledge and understanding of your specific situation. The opinions expressed in this book are those of the authors, or of those individuals quoted herein, and are based on their own personal experience. Other writers will undoubtedly offer conflicting opinions, which we encourage you to consider.

Now, with that out of the way, as you flip through this book, you'll notice right away that the majority of the photographs are not professionally done. They are not the best poses for the subjects; they are not airbrushed, nor are they altered in any way. In some cases, they are actually very amateurish. This is deliberate. We could have hired professional photographers to go out and make the individuals in these case studies look spectacular, especially in the "after" poses. Instead, we accepted the photos they offered us without any attempt to alter them. Most were taken by family members or nurses in a doctor's office.

We believe that showing you the "real" pictures allows you to clearly see the actual progress these band patients have made, but without any hype or exaggeration. You deserve to know what you're getting into, and to the best of our ability, we want to present you with the real picture—not something you'd see on a television commercial.

Most of our patients are thrilled with the adjustable gastric band, and for many it has led to spectacular results. But don't be fooled. There are trade-offs, lifestyle changes, and some cosmetic things that simply cannot be altered. That being said, it is our fondest desire that the personal stories and pictures contained in this book will offer you an element of hope, as they have for many others who have seen them.

Wishing you great losses,

Robert W. Sewell, M.D.,
and Linda Rohrbough

Introduction

How We Got Here

When one life is changed, the world is changed.
—Thomas L. Johns

Robert W. Sewell, M.D.'s Story:
Master® Laparoscopic Surgeon

I have to admit, I didn't exactly embrace "the band" when I first heard about it. It sounded like just another gimmick procedure, and I had a legitimate surgical practice and a decent reputation I'd spent 23 years building.

To provide some context for my involvement in the adjustable gastric band (AGB) phenomenon, it is important to understand that as a general surgeon, I spend most of my time operating within the abdomen. As you might imagine, performing abdominal operations on an extremely obese patient is much more difficult than operating on a thin patient. Dealing with the unyielding nature of fat stored in and around the abdomen often made me feel as if I'd done an hour or more of isometric exercises. For that reason, and for many years, I would say to anyone who would listen, "I hate fat!" At the same time I was always quick to add that, if I had the medical "Midas touch" to cure one disease, it would not be heart disease, diabetes, or even cancer; it would be obesity. My rationale was that if obesity were eliminated, many of those other illnesses would become far less common and easier to treat. Besides, my job as a surgeon would be easier.

In December of 1989, I witnessed my first laparoscopic gallbladder operation, and my perspective on abdominal surgery changed forever. It became clear to me that virtually any surgical operation could be done using a laparoscopic approach, which makes use of a small camera to look into the cavity, allowing intra-abdominal procedures to be performed without the need for large incisions. Since that day I have vigorously pursued these minimally invasive techniques, and today my entire practice is limited to such procedures.

While the benefits of the minimally invasive approach for the patient were obvious, a side benefit for me also became apparent. Carbon dioxide gas used to inflate the abdomen during laparoscopic surgery holds the abdominal wall up, and does it without physical effort from me or my assistants. All of a sudden operating on obese patients was more or less the same as operating on anybody else—no more "fighting the fat" just to get access to the inside of the abdomen.

Over the past 15 years, laparoscopic surgery has provided me with countless opportunities to be involved in a truly revolutionary process that is changing the entire field of general surgery. I have not only performed these new procedures but have been actively involved in training many of my colleagues in these innovative techniques. I've had the privilege of lecturing on this topic and supervising various laboratory sessions around the world. My motto was, If it's new ground-breaking technology, I want to be involved, both in performing and teaching the procedures—except for bariatric surgery.

The surgical treatment of obesity was a very sore subject in most surgical circles during the 1970s, when I was in training. The procedures I was aware of were fraught with serious complications and were considered fringe medicine by the vast majority of surgeons. I avoided surgical treatment for obesity like the plague. Actually, I was taught very little about obesity, except that it was more a personal lifestyle choice than an actual illness. I was taught to believe that obese people needed a psychiatrist, not a surgeon. So when I was approached about doing laparoscopic gastric bypass in the mid-1990s, I replied without hesitation, "No way. I am not getting involved in that."

In 2000, when I was first approached about the laparoscopic adjustable gastric band, I didn't exactly embrace it, either. It sounded like just another weight-loss gimmick, designed to take advantage of people desperately seeking a surgical solution to a psychological problem. I had a legitimate surgical practice and a good reputation, and I didn't want to jeopardize any of it by doing a procedure sure to be labeled as illegitimate by my peers. That all changed when I was approached by an oral surgeon colleague about advising a close personal friend of his. He told me that David, a prominent local businessman, wanted the band procedure and was looking for an experienced laparoscopic surgeon. I agreed to talk to David by phone and was actually planning to talk him out of the foolish idea.

During our discussion, David made a very compelling argument for getting a band. He had been overweight his entire adult life and had tried every diet I had ever heard of and several others I wasn't familiar with. I finally conceded he might be a candidate for the band, but then I told him that I didn't do the operation; however, a close friend and colleague of mine in Miami was doing the band operation. Needless to say, David was eager to make the contact.

By this time, my interest had been piqued. I realized that I didn't really know enough about the procedure to offer David any sound advice. I knew the band requires frequent follow-up visits and adjustments. And I was worried about the fact that, after surgery, David would be half a continent away from his surgeon. So I told David I was willing to provide his follow-up visits and his adjustments myself. I suggested that I'd be willing to go with him to Miami to watch his surgery in preparation for the follow-up work. It would also give me a chance to catch up with my friend, and get his insights on the band. It would also give me a chance to see for myself exactly how the procedure was done, so I could speak more intelligently about it in the future.

David made a quick trip to Miami to meet the surgeon, and he took his college-age daughter along. As it turned out, they were both candidates for the procedure, and both were scheduled to have the band operation less than a month later. When the time came for the trip to Miami, I was shocked to find that David had made arrangements for me and my nurse to fly from Dallas to Miami at his expense. First class, no less!

Both surgeries were performed the same day and were completed uneventfully. My colleague in Miami was very enthusiastic about the band. He and his partners had been part of the FDA trials during the previous two years, and they had done about 200 bands with very few complications and promising results. But, he admitted to me, he was doing far more gastric bypass operations, simply because insurance was not covering the band. I found that interesting, but not surprising.

When I saw David and his daughter back in my office about a week after their operations, they were both feeling well and offered no complaints. In fact they could barely contain their enthusiasm, based on the fact that they were already losing weight. After several adjustments and witnessing the clear evidence that the band was working for both father and daughter, I decided to get the required training to do the band myself. All of a sudden I became directly involved in exactly the type of practice I had vowed never to pursue. However, after seeing the excitement of those two people and remembering my career-long wish for the "Midas touch," I was convinced this was the right choice.

Through the training process and discussions with other surgeons, it was very clear that there was far more to an adjustable gastric band practice than just doing the surgery. Since that time, my practice has undergone a significant change. I still do all the same laparoscopic operations I did before, but about half of my patients now are adjustable gastric band patients. But the biggest change in my practice has been the development of a comprehensive weight management program in support of the band procedure.

Suffice it to say, caring for band patients has required a major reorganization in my approach to the practice of surgery. Traditionally, surgeons are more or less like firefighters—we're called in at times of crisis to extinguish a problem and then return to the firehouse. Except in very complicated cases, patients don't usually follow up with their surgeon more than a few times before being sent back to their primary doctor. As a result, most surgeons (and most patients) have a "fix-it and move on" attitude. That just doesn't apply to obesity or the adjustable gastric band.

Obesity is a chronic disease, and treatment with the band requires regular monitoring, periodic adjustments, and nearly continuous patient support in order to be successful. To accomplish this required me to make major modifications in my schedule, office personnel, and, most important, my practice philosophy. But, I have to say the results have greatly exceeded my expectations. Seeing the excitement in the eyes of patients who are finally achieving successful weight loss is far more rewarding than I ever imagined. As a result I undertook the task of writing this book along with one of my patients, who is a professional writer, in an effort to help shed some light on the problem of obesity and how the laparoscopic adjustable gastric band can be used to treat it successfully.

In the words of Hippocrates, "Extreme remedies are very appropriate for extreme diseases."

Linda Rohrbough's Story
AGB Patient and Award-Winning Author

When Dr. Sewell told me, "It's not your fault," I didn't believe him. Not because I didn't want to. I did. But lots of stuff went through my mind, and most of it had to do with my past failures and what I'd been programmed to believe.

I was not overweight until I got married. I remember when I was 16, I worked with a middle-aged, new mother on a church project. Every time I saw her, she just kept getting bigger and bigger. I thought with disgust, "Why can't she just stop eating?"

Two years later, several events occurred in my life. I was in a horseback riding accident and suffered a skull fracture that put me in the hospital for a week. Then I went through my high school graduation ceremony. And I got married two days later (an event my beloved and I had planned for four years—we met when I was 14 and he was 15). I started gaining weight in the hospital and barely fit into the wedding dress I'd bought months earlier. (And I'd tried that dress on every week except the one when I was in the hospital.)

After the wedding, my husband and I starved, literally. But we were too proud to let anyone know how much we struggled financially. I thought it was an aftereffect from the horseback riding accident that I didn't feel well enough to hang on to the job I had doing credit card processing on the swing shift; so I turned in my notice. My husband was working 14-hour days doing roofing. We were both miserable. To say I got plump would be an understatement.

I went to my family doctor. He asked me what I had for breakfast. When I said a piece of cake, he glared, got his nurse, and asked her to give me a diet plan—loudly enough for everyone in the waiting room to hear. I was so humiliated I didn't know what to say. But I stopped talking about it.

I was hungry all the time. I sat in our apartment in a bathrobe with the curtains drawn and cried. After a while, I got sick of that and decided to get a job. I remember walking into K-Mart; nothing fit but a size 18, when I used to wear a size 12. I sobbed uncontrollably in the dressing room for about 30 minutes, then went out and made my purchase.

I talked a local fabric store manager into hiring me and made model garments to have clothes to wear. I tried fasting and exercise, separately and in combination. I rode a bike. I worked two jobs at one point. Nothing helped.

I turned up pregnant a year later. Now that we were getting another life involved, my spouse and I packed what we could into our '66 Chevy II and went off to Kansas State University. We picked Kansas because out-of-state tuition there was cheaper than in-state tuition in Colorado.

It was at K-State that I found a diet program called "Stucky Points for Weight Control." With the help of the university dietitian, I lost 75 pounds in eight months. I was going to be their poster child. But I couldn't maintain. I ballooned up again, only the result was that I weighed more in a year and a half than before I'd started the diet. Even though my grade point average was 3.9, I felt like a failure.

And that was the story. Diet, weigh more, diet, weigh more. I experienced failure after failure, which only made the situation worse. I did not have the courage to talk to a doctor again for help. I watched people who did Weight Watchers® and Jenny Craig® lose weight then gain it back—plus, I couldn't afford a program like that. So I learned to shop the sales at Lane Bryant. A friend in college who was also overweight and I had a running joke about our "uniform." We each had two pairs of pants and two blouses and one pair of shoes that fit. We did a load of laundry every day so our "uniform" would be clean for the next day.

I remember the day a doctor said I was morbidly obese. I sensed the heat climbing my cheeks, and I found the floor tile pattern extremely interesting. I was careful not to let anyone see how upset I felt.

When my husband graduated college, we moved to Amarillo, Texas, and life was even more miserable for me. I went to college again, on grants and scholarships I'd earned, had two kids now, and was bigger than ever before. I noticed people I hardly knew would find a need to tell me how to lose weight, assuming I didn't know I had a problem. I had trouble fitting into booths in restaurants, struggled with seat belts, and was tired all the time.

I started writing about computers when my husband got a job in Los Angeles. Computer user groups asked me to write "how-to" articles about things I'd learned for their newsletters, and soon I was writing articles for national computer magazines. Before long I was working for an international computer news network.

It was in LA that I found the worst weight prejudice I've ever experienced. People, especially men, would yell obscenities at me about my weight when I was out walking. I still walked, but I felt a lot of fear. And I stopped trying to lose weight. I made the decision that I needed to accept the way I was—since I felt there wasn't anything I could do.

And I decided to enjoy food. As I got more successful writing, I worked on skills to help people look past my weight. I learned to make jokes, like "Fat people are jolly." On an airplane, I'd ask the stewardess for a seat belt extender and add, "And can you bring it so everyone can see you do it?" Airplanes were especially bad. The people who work for the airlines would often sigh and roll their eyes when they saw me coming. I figured it was because I weighed as much as two people and I was only paying for one. Often another passenger, whoever got stuck sitting next to me, was going to suffer as well. I'd drolly say to the wide-eyed, fear-filled face of the other passenger, as I shoe-horned myself into the seat, "Lucky you, getting to sit next to me." They'd usually chuckle.

I had a doctor tell me during a routine medical exam, "You know, you're extremely overweight."

I put my hands on my cheeks. "Oh no! What am I going to tell my family? What will my friends think?" The doctor just shook her head and left the room.

I had a friend say at least I kept myself clean. Another friend asked how I put up with the invasive things people said to me about my weight. I told her I was learning to accept myself.

At one point, I memorized all the Bible verses about obesity, thinking that might help. But they seemed contradictory. "The righteous will be made fat." And from Proverbs, "The drunkard and the glutton will come to poverty and drowsiness will clothe a man with rags."

When I started writing books, I became even more successful. I won three national awards for my writing. I thought my success might help my self-esteem, which in turn would help me lose weight. That didn't happen.

At the peak of my computer book writing, in 1998, I was in a car accident and suffered a broken back. I only thought I had been in pain before then. In the hospital, I was fitted with a body brace that the technician turned upside down because he said it wouldn't fit me right side up. I needed a heavy-duty wheelchair, and an oversized recliner became my bed. I was heavily medicated for a long time, learning to deal with constant agony. Over a period of two years I retrained myself to walk using a treadmill.

I heard the same thing over and over from the medical advisors I consulted during the course of my treatment: "This would be a lot easier if you could lose weight." I didn't say much, but I'd think, "It would be a lot easier if I could fly, too." But I realized I needed to do something, so I started attending programs and seminars to teach me how to improve my self-esteem.

It wasn't too long after I could get around again that I met someone from Overeaters Anonymous who'd lost more than 100 pounds. So I started going to OA meetings. I listened and envied the bulimics and the ones who'd figured out how to conquer their bodies. At this time we lived in Dallas, and my husband had excellent medical insurance. My beloved is overweight, too, but I was bigger; he told me he was struggling with embarrassment over my appearance.

On a routine visit to my doctor for a checkup, the nurse weighing me took the scale to the max, where it clunked. It only went to 350 pounds. She shrugged and said, "Oh well," before she led me off to a treatment room. I knew that meant I wasn't close to 350. I was probably a good deal over.

I took a risk and talked to the doctor about my weight. He said I needed a lifestyle change. I told him I was walking, and he said, "People who are practically dead can walk. Just visit an old folk's home and watch them roam up and down the halls." He told me to drink more water, suggesting that I work my way up to 100 ounces a day.

The lifestyle change idea stuck in my head. I started watching thin people and noticed that many of them carried a bottle of water. Over a period of two years, I dropped soft drinks and worked up to drinking 100 ounces of water a day. And during that time, I got down to 335 pounds. Clearly, this wasn't anything to write home about. While the scale was going in a better direction, it wasn't enough.

I started checking into weight loss surgery. My husband's office moved, and so we relocated to the other side of DFW, north of Ft. Worth. I looked for a new doctor. By this time I was on medication for high blood pressure. I was also taking a number of vitamin supplements I'd discovered through research or friends, with the goal of feeling better. I found a new doctor, and she became very proactive in my care. She put me in touch with a physical therapist who started helping me deal with the pain in my back and knees. He prescribed orthotics for my shoes, along with exercises. He treated me about three days a week to help me beat the pain, and it was working.

As we became friends, I confided I'd given up on losing weight. He told me about some surgical options, some of which I'd already checked out. But he knew about a new product, the adjustable gastric band. He explained to me how it worked and told me he'd worked with gastric bypass patients and AGB, or "band," patients. Of the two, he said the band people didn't seem to have problems, and they kept the weight off. I told him that surgery scared me. I don't think I'll ever forget what he said. He was on a stool, working on my leg, and he stopped, placed his hand on my knee, looked me in the eye, and said, "Linda, if I were in your position, I'd do it."

Later that same day he faxed me an ad for Robert W. Sewell, M.D. It said, "Step Out of the Shadow of Obesity." I called and was told about a free seminar Doc offered, so I signed up. I told the OA group about my plans. They weren't totally discouraging, but I could tell that they generally frowned on what I was considering. The OA literature said surgery was in the same category as throwing up after eating. I nearly canceled going to Doc's seminar several times. When I did go, I was late and sat in the back.

I missed the first part of the presentation, but then they introduced Don, whose story you'll read later on. Don, a professional public speaker, was talking as he walked past me from the back of the room. They showed videos of Don before the surgery. With his characteristic dark bow-tie, he looked like Humpty-Dumpty. When he got to the front, he showed us the belt he used to wear. I thought two people could wear the belt at the same time. Afterward, he took time with me one-on-one to answer my questions about OA, which he also had attended. Don at that time was down over 100 pounds, with 100 to go. But he was happy, looked healthy, and was obviously successful both in his weight loss and his profession.

I felt hope so strong in my chest it hurt. I made an appointment for consultation with Dr. Sewell. I weighed in at 331 the day I talked to him in his office. I was afraid. Failing again was almost more than I could take. After he explained to me how the AGB worked, I went out to discuss the financial details with Sue, his administrator. Sue is a very compassionate person, and I found my eyes filled with tears. She said, "Are you all right?"

I got a grip and managed to get out the words, "I'm scared."

She said, "How about if I have one of the other band patients call you?"

On the way home, I had all kinds of doubts going through my head. Could I make this change? This band doesn't work for everyone; would it work for me? What did the psychological evaluation mean, and what if I couldn't get through it? And what if I couldn't keep the weight off? What if this problem was some character flaw of mine?

Sue was as good as her word. When I arrived home there was a message on my answering machine from Gayle, another band patient who helps in the mentoring program for Dr. Sewell. She was charming and funny. She answered all my questions and then said, "Do you want to see me eat?"

Boy, did I. We made a lunch date. Her daughter came along, and they both answered my questions. I watched Gayle eat and I was sold. She wouldn't even let me pay for lunch. Gayle was lovely, down to a size 6 in her 5-foot, 2-inch frame from a 26/28 a year earlier. She showed me her "before" photos, but it was still hard to imagine her with an extra 80 pounds. She, too, was another professionally successful woman.

When I heard about Dr. Sewell's pre-op diet, I wondered if I'd have the self-discipline to carry it off. I was asked to have a protein shake for breakfast, one for lunch, and a salad or vegetables with four ounces of lean beef or chicken and low-fat dressing for dinner. I lived on McDonald's grilled chicken Caesar salads. I was miserable.

Meanwhile, what was supposed to be a three-week pre-op diet turned into a seven-week marathon. I was scheduled for surgery in the middle of December of 2003, but we couldn't get the insurance approval. So I ended up doing the pre-op diet from December 2 until January 19. I was so hungry all the time, I felt I was starving. But with the encouragement of Dr. Sewell's staff and especially his nurse, Stacie, I stayed with it. I weighed daily at first, but I stopped after a while. Did it matter, I asked myself? I was doing what I needed to do to shrink my liver. If I lost weight, fine, but I didn't want to discourage myself.

When I came in to weigh just before surgery, I was down a whopping 27 pounds. I currently hold the record with Dr. Sewell's patients for the most weight lost pre-op.

Gayle came to see me both before and after surgery, and my family stayed with me, too. Doc found a hernia (I suspect that was another leftover from the car accident) and repaired it, along with placing the band. So my recovery was longer than that of most band patients.

Today, as I write this in April 2007, I've lost 136 pounds since December of 2003, which is when I started the pre-op diet. Don't get me wrong, it's not that there aren't challenges. There are. I've learned pretty fast what I can and cannot eat. And if I attempt to overeat, I throw up, which I hate. I've had to learn to eat very small, pencil-eraser size bites of food and chew it very well. I carefully watch my water intake, making sure I get plenty so I don't get dehydrated. I monitor my protein intake as well.

But I'm off the blood pressure medicine, and the orthotics are out of my shoes. The smallest size I can wear now is a 12, when I used to wear a size 32. I was measured at a year from my pre-op evaluation and have lost a total of 55 inches. Airplanes now feel roomy, and the seatbelts are way too big. I can cross my legs. I get out of a chair without any preparation or pain. My back doesn't hurt. I walk the mall with ease. My knees don't hurt. I shop at GAP, Old Navy, and Chicos, places I'd never even dared to go into before. I can buy jeans at Wal-Mart. I exercise (yoga and bike riding under the supervision of an exercise therapist), and I see a psychologist to help me adjust to the positive changes in my life.

One of the biggest changes was, when I got down 40 pounds, people started asking me to work for them. I never had that happen before, and it's still a little scary. I'm used to selling myself, and I don't have to do that anymore.

Do I do this band thing perfectly? Hardly, but I'm getting better at making working choices for myself. The cool thing is that I don't have to be perfect. I can screw up, and the band keeps me on the wagon. I've gained a pound or two here and there, but that usually precipitates a large weight drop of several pounds.

Further, I save more than $700 a month, an unexpected bonus. I no longer have insurance copayments for the physical therapist or the blood pressure medicine. People say I eat like a bird, and my clothes cost a lot less. Pretty amazing.

Would I recommend the band? In a heartbeat. I know now that obesity really wasn't my fault, and it's not your fault either. But the band is not an answer that comes without effort or education. That's what this book is about.

SECTION 1

Obesity in Our Culture

Obesity

The Great American Health Problem

Reality is something you rise above.
—Liza Minelli

One of the most basic of human activities has been the pursuit of food. In its most primitive form, this involved hunting wild animals or searching for edible plants. Throughout the millennia, finding enough to eat has often been difficult. Wars have been fought over fertile tracts of land or abundant hunting grounds, often on empty stomachs. The story of Joseph in the Book of Genesis typifies the struggles man has experienced throughout recorded history.

Joseph was a servant who was elevated to second in command of all Egypt because he was able to interpret the pharaoh's recurring dream. In that dream he saw seven fat cows and seven thin cows, which Joseph correctly interpreted as a sign that there would be seven years of plentiful crops followed by seven years of drought and failed crops. This information was used by Joseph, the pharaoh's chosen overseer of the entire nation, to store up grain for future use and avoid the cycle of famine that was common in those days. This story obviously revolves around food, and it speaks volumes about the relationship between food, political power, and social status.

The domestication of livestock and raising of crops are a hallmark of our modern civilization. With the Industrial Revolution came improved farming techniques with more abundant crops and larger herds of cattle and other livestock, raised specifically as food. Just as important was the development of a transportation system capable of bringing that food to a hungry market. The benefits of these advances were obvious. Compared with just 100 years ago, U.S. industry has achieved an unprecedented command over the feeding of an entire population. At no time in recorded history, except perhaps in the Garden of Eden, has food been more plentiful, at a lower cost.

In the 1970s, the stated objective of our society was to wipe out world hunger. That is not only an admirable goal, but today it even seems achievable. However, in recent years we have witnessed a serious side effect of the pursuit of that goal. This "land of plenty" has become a nation of overweight and obese individuals. While many are quick to point a blaming finger at the "fat" man or woman on the street, the problem is much more complex. Obesity is a disease with its roots in human physiology and is greatly influenced by our environment.

Our Relationship with Food
G. Dick Miller, Psychologist

If you look at recent history, my parents, the World War II generation, had a garden no matter what. Because for them as kids, the thing they had to have was food. They stored potatoes and apples for winter, and my Dad still does that, even though he can buy whatever he wants.

Our attitude as a society has changed. We fast, we feast. We no longer think of food as a necessity. Few people in this country know anyone who is going hungry. But we know a lot of people who have weight problems. Part of the reason is that our lifestyle no longer demands physical labor to get the food we eat.

But it's more than abundance without exercise. We're pressured socially. Most places I visit, I'm asked, "Can I get you something?" Or they'll say, "You've got to be hungry, you've traveled all this way." People find themselves uncomfortable with me if I don't eat their food. If I don't eat, I hear, "Is something wrong with the food? Do you want to go someplace else? Why didn't you eat all of it?"

In addition to social pressure, we're enticed. Look at what advertising agencies do to attract us by associating food with music. I met a guy who works for the company that developed the drink Fango Tango. No one could remember the first Fango Tango jingle, but I did. After I sang the song for him, I could taste Fango Tango. Think about how powerful that is, especially knowing I first heard the song in 1954—a whopping 52 years ago.

Movie theaters have done something similar using smell. I hardly ever eat popcorn except in a movie theater. But once I'm there and get a whiff of popcorn, even though I know I'm going to eat after the movie, I get uncomfortable and feel I must have some.

It's common to use the word "love" when we talk about provisions. A few generations ago people talked about "sweet-tasting" corn. Now we "love" the corn. We talk about food the way characters talk about each other in a romance novel, in hushed tones, with great anticipation. I said all that to say we have a love/hate relationship with food, and it's affecting our waistlines.

The human body is designed to allow excess food energy to be stored as fat for later use. It is our safety net in the event of famine. This process has helped preserve our species throughout the ages when the availability of food was in question. However, when a shortage never comes, the fat stores continue to increase. Obesity has been known to exist throughout history, even in ancient times, but prior to the last half of the twentieth century it was actually quite rare. Today obesity is an epidemic in the United States and, to a lesser extent, throughout Western civilization. It affects all ages, without regard to gender, race, ethnic background, or socioeconomic status.

In 2004, approximately two-thirds of U.S. adults were overweight. What's more, we know it. Dieting has become "the great American pastime," and is a multibillion-dollar industry. We are also told how important it is to exercise. Fitness centers are everywhere these days and will gladly get you started, with or without supervision. The "home-gym" is also a hot seller, especially around the first of the year, when we ceremonially vow to start working out to shed those unwanted pounds. Despite all these efforts, the problem is actually getting measurably worse. We must be missing something. What can be done to successfully combat this nemesis?

To begin to answer the question of obesity, it is important first to quantify the problem. While most Americans are overweight, the term "obese" is actually a medical term that implies a specific degree of excess weight. But weight alone doesn't tell the whole story. An individual's height obviously must be taken into consideration. A person who is 6 foot, 6 inches and weighs 250 pounds is not particularly overweight, but someone at the same weight who is 5 foot, 3 inches is morbidly obese. Both height and weight are used to calculate what is called the Body Mass Index, or BMI. A BMI is calculated by taking the person's weight in kilograms divided by their height in meters squared ($BMI = kg/m^2$).

A normal BMI is between 20 and 25 kg/m^2, while obesity is defined as between 30 and 40 kg/m^2. If the BMI is over 40 kg/m^2, the condition is known as morbid obesity. Morbid obesity is widely defined as being 100 pounds or more overweight. For purposes of simplicity throughout the remainder of this book I will drop the kg/m^2 and just use the designation BMI when referring to Body Mass Index.

In my example, the 6-foot, 6-inch person weighing 250 has a BMI of 28.9, while the 5-foot, 3-inch person has a BMI of 44.9. There is a Body Mass Index table in the Resources chapter (page 262) at the end of the book for your convenience in determining your own BMI. Below is a table showing the BMI categories along with the related risk of other disease for each BMI range and associated waist size.

Obesity is clearly a major healthcare problem because of its direct causative relationship to a number of serious health problems, including Type 2 diabetes, hypertension, heart disease, and cancer. The incidence of adult onset diabetes has skyrocketed in the last decade, and the healthcare costs associated with diabetes have jumped as well. The American Diabetes Association estimated that the direct and indirect expense associated with diabetes in the United States was $123 billion in 2002. That was an increase of 27 percent compared with just five years earlier.

Despite the obvious relationship between obesity and a number of major health problems, medical science has had little to offer the obese patient other than medications designed to curb the appetite. Some of these drugs have shown promise, but most have been plagued either by significant side effects or a lack of effectiveness. There is currently some optimism surrounding emerging hormone therapies and even genetic manipulation, but these experimental technologies have yet to be proven. In the absence of effective treat-

Risk of Associated Disease according to BMI and Waist Size

BMI		Waist less than or equal to 40 in. (men) or 35 in. (women)	Waist greater than 40 in. (men) or 35 in. (women)
18.5 or less	Underweight	—	N/A
18.5–24.9	Normal	—	N/A
25.0–29.9	Overweight	Increased	High
30.0–34.9	Obese	High	Very High
35.0–39.9	Obese	Very High	Very High
40 or greater	Extremely (Morbid) Obese	Extremely High	Extremely High

Source: Partnership for Healthy Weight Management, www.consumer.gov/weightloss/bmi.htm.

ments for obesity, physicians are currently left with a variety of medications designed to treat merely the chronic symptoms of the disease, such as diabetes, hypertension, and high cholesterol. While generally effective at controlling these secondary problems, the medications are often expensive, and most have side effects. More important, they don't do anything about the basic cause, obesity.

In keeping with our fast-paced lifestyle, many obese people are seeking a "quick fix" to their problem. After all, the "makeover" programs on television take the process of totally changing your appearance and make it look so simple. It all takes place in about an hour. What better way to get rid of those unwanted pounds than to have them surgically removed? Uninformed patients often consider liposuction and other body contouring procedures as weight management tools and are shocked to find following such procedures that they have lost only a few pounds. Such cosmetic procedures were never intended to achieve weight loss.

There are surgical operations designed specifically to promote weight loss. These procedures, known as bariatric surgery, typically rearrange the gastrointestinal tract and can have dramatic results. In recent years, bariatric surgical procedures have received tremendous media attention as treatment for morbid obesity.

The National Institutes of Health (NIH) reported in their 1991 consensus statement that the only treatment shown to be effective in the treatment of morbid obesity long-term is surgery. But the risks of the surgical procedures in use at the time the NIH made that statement are high, and recurrent weight gain has been more common than had been hoped. The numbers indicate that 1 in 100 gastric bypass surgery patients will die within a month of surgery. Five out of 100 will die within a year, and another 20 percent or more will be rehospitalized for complications related directly to their surgery. Despite the risk, the number of obesity operations has increased dramatically in recent years.

The lack of a safe and effective treatment option has many obese individuals feeling trapped. Dieting and exercise have not worked for them, and the risk of bariatric surgical procedures has made that option unacceptable to the majority of potential patients. Their frustration is usually compounded by the fact that most morbidly obese people are also suffering from one or more associated health problems. The perpetual treatment of their diabetes; high blood pressure; knee, hip, and back problems; acid reflux; or other weight-related conditions is not only exasperating but also costly.

Stephen's Story

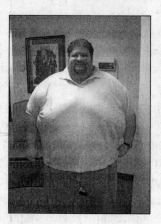
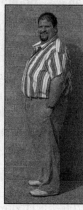

(Left) Stephen pre-op, 568 pounds.

(Right) Stephen, 17 months post-op, 362 pounds.

In the beginning, I was against band surgery. I kept telling myself I can do this, I can do it on my own. I was afraid of being put to sleep for surgery because, in my case, the odds were pretty good I would never wake up. I had no idea how much I weighed before I came to Dr. Sewell because most doctors' scales went up to only 350 pounds. When I weighed in at 568, I just cried and cried.

What changed my mind about the surgery was watching my sister and my mom, who both have the band—especially my sister. She started at close to 400 pounds and lost 80 with the band.

Initially, Dr. Sewell told me I had to lose weight before he'd do the surgery. I lost some, but I couldn't lose the amount needed. Then he told me there were other people with a higher BMI than mine who got the band, and he thought he could do it. He expected to be three to four hours in surgery, but after 45 minutes he was done. I was the first of his patients to get the larger 9cc band. That was May 12 of 2004.

Now, 17 months later, I've lost 206 pounds. It's the greatest thing I've ever done. I love it that Dr. Sewell says this is permanent and it'll be there the rest of my life.

I work out hard with weights and I do cardio. I realize the band is not going to be the cure-all, and you've got to add some exercise. I've heard every pound you lose is 2 pounds of pressure off your joints. I have very bad knees—no cartilage in one knee, and I've had two knee surgeries. Now with my weight loss, my knees feel so much better.

I see other changes already. We've gone to Disney World three years in a row, and usually I had to park myself somewhere and watch the world go by. One of the hardest things was when people used to ask to have their pictures taken with me because I'm so big. I noticed this time I walked past a group of kids and they didn't all turn around. Some did, but not all of them like they used to. And I was step for step with everyone during the three days. In addition, I recently did a 5K walk and passed people on the course. I feel great that I can put on a seatbelt in a car.

As for living with the band, I'm a firm believer in not drinking for two hours after I eat. I used to go into a restaurant and tell the waiter to bring me a pitcher. Not now.

I've been real lucky. Even at 568, I had people who supported me and could see positives in me. My older sister, who doesn't have a band, is my workout buddy along with her husband. She has always seen in me what I couldn't see in myself, and she told me I'd find a way to get the weight off.

Where I work, two people died after the gastric bypass. I work with only 200 people, so two deaths is a lot. In my family, three people have been banded, and we're all doing fine.

With severe sleep apnea, I sleep with a machine. But I notice my breathing is easier. I don't snore at all, and I don't wake until my alarm goes off. I used to wake up 30 to 40 times each night.

The worst thing for me in the beginning was people's perceptions. At six weeks after surgery, people were saying, "Are you still eating all that?" or "You've only lost 12 pounds?" I didn't put this on overnight, and I'm not going to take it off overnight, either.

My wife is my support. She loved me at my worst in my life. I cannot wait to be the husband I always wanted to be for her. I used to be very athletic, and I want to be that way again. I've been sterile, but I want to be able to have children. There's a chance I could be sterile because of my weight. We checked into adoption, but no agency will consider someone who is 35 years old and weighs over 500 pounds. They just don't think I'll live long enough to see the child grow up.

My next goal is to get to 250. When that happens, my wife says she's going to buy me a motorcycle.

The focus of this book is an innovative treatment that combines a much lower-risk, minimally invasive surgical procedure with a diet and exercise program. The adjustable gastric band was introduced in Belgium in 1992 and has enjoyed considerable popularity in the management of morbid obesity throughout the world. It received approval by the Federal Food and Drug Administration for use in the United States in June of 2002, following several years of clinical trials. By the end of 2003 more than 100,000 bands had been placed worldwide, with about 25,000 in the United States.

While the adjustable gastric band is providing considerable help to a number of morbidly obese individuals, it is not a panacea. Subsequent sections of this book endeavor to offer as much information as possible about this treatment, so anyone who is contemplating weight-loss surgery can make an educated and fully informed decision.

Why Dieting and Exercise Don't Work

*Every man has a right to his opinion,
but no man has a right to be wrong in his facts.*
— Bernard Baruch

Let's face it. Trying to lose weight is tough. If it were simple, you wouldn't be reading this book, right? On the other hand, for most of us, gaining weight is very easy. The reasons are as varied as are our personalities, but suffice it to say that readily available, high-calorie foods and a sedentary lifestyle lead the list of causes for obesity. Most of us eat way too much of the wrong things, and we get little or no exercise. The answer to the obesity epidemic is simple. You've heard it a million times: "Eat less, make better food choices, and get some exercise."

I have yet to meet an obese person who hasn't tried to follow that advice. Most have been on every available diet program, usually more than once. They have learned that to be successful takes tremendous discipline, which must be maintained over an extended period of time. That is especially true for those trying to lose large amounts of weight. Not surprisingly, most people are unable to sustain such an effort beyond just a few weeks or perhaps a couple of months, despite their best intentions.

Virtually all diets call for the individual to control not only what kind of food they eat but also to minimize the size of their portions. Such dietary restrictions almost always lead to hunger, and, sooner or later, it's profound hunger that becomes the undoing of the diet. When your stomach is growling and you can't think of anything but what you might find in the pantry or the refrigerator, willpower is simply not enough. Most people abandon their diet, not because they aren't getting results, but because they feel like they are starving. Once they are "off the wagon" the result is fairly predictable. The weight lost is quickly regained, plus a few extra pounds. Eventually another diet comes along, another commitment is made: "This time I know I can do it." The cycle of gaining and losing and regaining weight, called "yo-yoing," tends to be repeated over and over. Interestingly, "yo-yo" dieting also tends to slow down a person's overall metabolic rate, making future weight loss even more difficult.

The Physical and Psychological Links to Obesity
G. Dick Miller, Psychologist

I talked about the shift in attitudes from food as a necessity to something we have a relationship with. But there's also a physiological component, an evolution that's happened over the years. Psychologist Carl Jung said we have this collective unconscious—generations of attitudes, behaviors, and beliefs that now have become biology. With eating it plays out like this. We've had an abundance of food, and our children are now born with more fat cells. These cells create cravings, and they get priority treatment. As a consequence, our brains are bombarded, through the relationship between our hypothalamus gland and the fat cells, with demands for more and more chow.

I've seen this evolution and felt powerless to stop it. Early in my practice, I worked with weight-loss clients. But after a while it became obvious to me why I wasn't successful with people who came to me for weight management. Once someone was heavy enough that their metabolism changed, given everything against them, it was over. That's why the failure rate with diets is 95 percent. No matter how much I worked to help someone change their thinking and develop new coping skills, I couldn't keep them out of the environment long enough to get them to change. People need about nine months for their new thinking to take hold and their body chemistry to change. And I could not recommend the gastric bypass because I knew the mortality rate and the risk to the bypass patient's internal organs. Consequently, I stopped accepting weight management clients.

That is, until I found out about the AGB. The band is the best "library card" I've ever seen to get someone into the place where they can change. As Dr. Sewell says, the band is a tool. But it can be circumvented. AGB patients can make ice cream a beverage. And they'll do just that if they don't change their thinking and learn a new set of coping skills.

It is the change in our relationship with and our thinking about food that makes weight management work. If we change our thinking, we'll change our lifestyles and we'll change our results. The AGB is the first step in the process.

It is obvious that dieting has become big business. Whenever someone comes on television with their story of how they lost 30 or 40 pounds in six to eight weeks, it is always followed by the phrase "and so can you!" Americans spend more than $30 billion each year on diets and dietary products, yet dieting failures are the rule, not the exception. Such failures frequently lead to feelings of guilt and even depression, which can result in eating binges and even more weight gain. The negative effects on self-esteem are often compounded by all the publicity surrounding the so-called success stories. The fact is that, after numerous failures, some people just give up dieting and resign themselves to a life of being uncomfortably overweight.

So what about exercise? Without a doubt most Americans don't get enough exercise. Our everyday lives have been made much easier by the multitude of modern conveniences we take for granted. They have taken away much of what used to be required physical effort. Certainly, some people still have physically demanding jobs, but for many others it is now possible to work from home, shop from home, and, most important, even order dinner delivered. For those times when we do get out of the house we typically jump in the car and drive, even if we are going only a couple of blocks. The result is we use up very few calories as we go through our usual daily activities. Combine this lack of exercise with immediately available, high-calorie foods, brought to your door or picked up at the convenient drive-through, and the recipe for fattening America is complete.

Intuitively, almost everyone understands they need to get some exercise if they expect to shed those excess pounds. Witness the fact that over the past 30 years Americans have joined health and fitness clubs and hired personal trainers in record numbers. We have purchased countless pieces of home exercise equipment in an effort to make it easier and more convenient to get some exercise. But, during that same time, we have become increasingly overweight as a society.

The problem is that physically demanding activities are simply not part of our normal day-to-day life. They represent "extra" activities, which have no direct financial or social benefit for those who are chasing the American Dream. For many of us, exercise is an activity that takes up valuable time—time we don't have to spare. Hours spent working out can't be used to pick up the laundry or help the kids with their homework. That time isn't available to make a sales call, or clear out the paperwork piling up on the desk, or return that growing list of e-mail messages. How many times have you said, "I don't have time; I'll start tomorrow. I promise"?

Don's Story

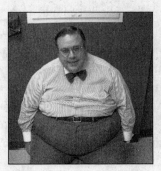 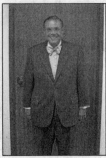

(Left) Don, pre-op, 385 pounds.

(Right) Don, two years post-op, 182 pounds.

I'm a lifetime fatty. As a cub scout, I had a 32-inch waist. I spent my entire adult life weighing between 300 and 400 pounds. I fly a lot and often first class. I was flying first class on an international trip and had to move to coach where I could get the arm rest up so I could use two seats. If I ever write a book about my weight loss, I plan to call it, "Too Fat for First Class."

I've lost 100 pounds or more on five different occasions. For example, I got involved in Overeaters Anonymous (OA) and lost 165 pounds—went from 320 to 156. I tried a liquid protein diet and lost 100 pounds. I did both Atkins and OA and made it from 435 down to 280.

I'm a researcher by trade. About the time Al Roker's gastric bypass hit the news I started researching weight-loss surgery. I checked out over 500 websites. I went to six public seminars and interviewed four surgeons.

My decision was motivated by three issues: geography, recovery time (because of my hectic schedule), and, most important, the reputation of the surgeon. I found Dr. Sewell through one of the guys in my Rotary club and began to explore his reputation with other doctors I knew. What a lot of people don't realize is that other surgeons who come across cases they feel are too risky to handle turn those cases over to Dr. Sewell. One doctor said to me that for laparoscopic surgery what you want is a great cutter, and Dr. Sewell is a great cutter.

I got my band on February 3, 2003. Pre-op I weighed in at 385. I've currently lost over 200 pounds. There have been some stumbles along the way. Dr. Sewell's never been real happy with me, because I've used a calorie methodology, meaning I try to keep my calorie intake low. So I didn't have that first adjustment for four to five months. I see the band as a device that keeps me from overeating. I've never had any real hunger pains. But I know Dr. Sewell would prefer I let the band do some of the work and that I lose more slowly.

Statistically, 50 percent of the people who go through weight-loss surgery end up having some type of plastic surgery. I'm into body sculpting. On March 4, 2004, I had a nine-hour surgery in which the plastic surgeon took off a strip of skin 12 inches wide all the way around my middle. I went in at 201 pounds expecting to weigh a lot less than 200 when I came out.

But I was dehydrated, so they ended up giving me 14 liters of fluid and I came out weighing 225. However, after healing, I lost 8 inches off my waist, so I made it into a size 38 pant. I was in a size 48 pre-op. I've had less extensive plastic surgery since then, including operations to take care of the other hanging skin areas on my legs, chest, neck, and so forth. It looks like I'll have four plastic surgeries all together before I'm done.

I have a couple of observations about my weight loss. One is I'm cold all the time. When you get on the Internet, you hear that complaint often from people who have lost a lot of weight. I talked to a neurologist about it, and she said it will take my body a couple of years to adjust to the new me. I also notice that my weight fluctuates. My lowest weight was 182 pounds, but I tend to be somewhere between that and 210, depending on how hard I work on my food choices. Right now I'm at 208.

I also feel that my interpersonal relationships were based on weight and that my personality was shaped by it. I'm a pure "Type A" personality, and I felt I spent my life compensating. I was the fat man, so I had to prove myself. Now everyone says I'm easier to live with. I'm softer, more mellow. I do know I like myself more.

One more thing I want to add is that my income has more than doubled since I lost the weight. There are fat bigots out there and prejudice. When I lost the weight, I generated a lot of successful energy from relationships without expending any extra effort. The weight is no longer an encumbrance.

Consequently, my income, which was already extremely good, is just blowing out. I have more than recovered the money I spent on the band and plastic surgeries with my increased income, meaning that the surgeries have more than paid for themselves. Now that I'm a normal looking corporate type, I realize how much the weight was holding me back. I removed a major barrier to my career advancement when I got banded, and I feel terrific about that. So the way I see it, the band has a strong potential economic payoff.

For those who are extremely overweight, exercise can present an entirely different set of problems. Someone who is carrying around an extra 75 pounds or more may find that physical activity of any type is difficult or impossible because of pain or immobility. That is particularly true as obese people grow older. The chronic burden of obesity on the back, hips, knees, ankles, and feet frequently results in significant pain with even limited exercise. Even if their joints don't hurt, just gathering the energy to get started in a regular exercise program can present a major obstacle. Exercising is not an option for those who become short of breath just walking from the car into the house.

For those who can participate in a regular exercise program, the results are frequently far less than what they expected. Increasing physical activity alone often doesn't lead to sustainable weight loss. It must be combined with a reasonable dietary plan. The irony is that exercising may actually have the effect of increasing a person's appetite. Hunger becomes a particularly difficult problem following a workout, and it is easy to rationalize an extra snack or a large order of fries as a fitting reward for all the hard work. However, the truth is that a candy bar or a milkshake contains more calories than most people can burn off walking for an hour on a treadmill.

Pat's Story

My internist, who'd been my doctor since 1980, said, "I'm going to fire you as a patient." He proceeded to tell me that my diabetes had progressed to the place where he estimated I had only a year to live. He then said, "You haven't listened to me in 25 years, and I'm not going to sit here and watch myself lose you."

I was shocked. We'd been friends, and I could tell he was upset, too. I asked for more time, and he repeated that he'd already given me a quarter of a century. So I asked for another three months.

I left his office knowing I had to do something about my weight. But what to do? I went to another doctor about cysts and tumors in my breasts, and I asked him about the gastric bypass. He thought it was an "abortion to your body." I told him the internist was going to quit me. He mentioned the band and Dr. Sewell. I talked to my daughter-in-law, who was a nursing student at Texas Christian University (TCU), and she also gave me Dr. Sewell's contact information. I called, found out about a free informational seminar he was having, and drove two hours with my husband to attend.

At the seminar I decided to do this, and my husband was on board. Dr. Sewell had a patient there who was delightful, a young, attractive, vivacious person. I asked her, "Can you have Coke®?" and she said, "Yes, if you let it go flat." Someone asked if she could have a big steak, and I thought she was very honest when she said no. But you know, I have found, while those things were important to me then, they're not important anymore.

I was turned down by my insurance three times, but I kept fighting. I was going to get a band and would have paid for it myself. As it turns out, I was on the pre-op diet two months and doing very well—really losing. So I said to myself, "Why am I doing surgery if I'm losing on the pre-op diet?" Then I answered myself, "Because I'll gain it back if I put a cracker in my mouth." I went back to my internist during the pre-op diet, and since I'd lost weight, he said he'd stick it out for six more months.

I'm 5 feet, 4 inches, and started at 265 pounds. Now, two years out, I fluctuate between 125 and 130 pounds. I feel wonderful. I used to have headaches if I didn't eat, and I took massive doses of Advil®. Since the band surgery, I've taken Tylenol® only 10 times in two years. I had leg problems that have mostly disappeared. A year and a half ago I fell, pulled ligaments in my right leg, and was in the emergency room. My internist, who is still my doctor, by the way, said, "Do you realize with the fall you took, had you not lost weight, you'd be in a wheel chair for the rest of your life?" I don't even limp now, and I was in physical therapy for six weeks.

It's like I can't say enough. What can you say about people who saved your life? Someone asked me when I was going to have the band removed, and I said, "Never." I'll tell anyone about the band who'll stand still long enough to listen. In fact, sometimes I find myself chasing someone down the hall at work, saying, "There's just one more thing."

Despite all the problems that plague dieting and exercise, those two activities remain the basis for any sustainable weight-loss program. It is mandatory to control both the amount and the types of foods that are consumed to ensure adequate nutrition while decreasing total weight. Likewise, regular physical exercise not only improves the function of heart and lungs, it also increases the body's basal metabolic rate. That means people who work out regularly burn more calories, even at rest, than those who don't exercise.

Given all the positive things that can come from a good diet and a regular exercise program, it would seem that everyone should be eager to participate—and most of us are—but only to a point. Right or wrong, we live in a society based on immediate gratification and increasing creature comforts. When viewed in that context, dieting is often seen as simply depriving ourselves of what we want and deserve, and exercising just for the sake of working up a sweat is not any fun. As a result, participation in dieting and exercise is for many only a half-hearted effort. What we are really looking for is an immediate effect with minimal inconvenience and a guaranteed result. That is the way we have been programmed to think, but it isn't the way our bodies work. In the next few chapters we'll explore more of this "quick fix" concept for treating obesity, and why such options often fail.

Causes and Treatments of Obesity

3

How the Digestive System Functions

The trouble with people is not that they don't know but that they know so much that ain't so.

—Josh Billings, *Josh Billings's Encyclopedia of Wit and Wisdom*

There is an old saying: "You are what you eat." But, obviously, if all you eat is vegetables, you don't become a vegetable. Everything we eat undergoes a complex process inside our bodies called digestion, which is a fundamental part of sustaining life. In order to understand the problem of obesity and also how various weight-loss operations work, it is important to have a basic knowledge of how our digestive system works.

All of the building blocks and vital sources of energy our bodies use are contained within the food we eat. Digestion can be summed up as the process of changing food both physically and chemically, all the way down to the molecular level. The hamburger you had for lunch must be broken down into its molecular components before any of it can be absorbed into your bloodstream. It is only then that the carbohydrates, fats, and proteins we ingest can actually be used by the body.

The digestive system breaks down proteins into amino acids, carbohydrates into simple sugars, and fats into fatty acids and other molecules such as cholesterol and triglycerides. These basic building blocks are then used either as sources of energy or as structural elements for growing new tissues, repairing injured areas, or restoring parts that wear out naturally. Anything not needed to meet immediate needs is eventually converted into fat and stored in various areas throughout the body for future use.

The Digestive System

The human digestive system is composed of two basic parts, as shown in the figure below. The main component is the long tube that begins at the mouth and ends at the anus and is called the alimentary tract. The rest of the system is composed of organs that add various chemicals essential for digestion into the alimentary tract. These include the salivary glands, the liver, and the pancreas.

The system seems fairly simple. You put food in one end, and eventually the waste material comes out the other. However, what goes on in between is one of the true wonders of life. Whether the individual is a world-class athlete or a newborn baby, a manual laborer or a grandmother in a rocking chair, each body requires the same nutrients and gets them in the same way. We eat to live.

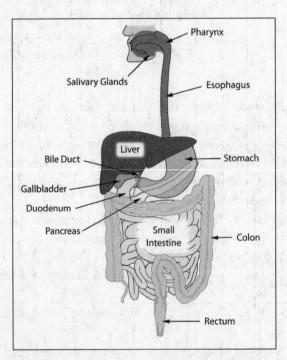

The digestive system is composed of two basic parts: the alimentary tract, which is the tube from the mouth to the anus, and a number of organs that add various chemicals for digestion.

Mechanical Digestion

The voluntary process of eating initiates a complex cascade of events that occur automatically. You might think this process doesn't begin until you put food into your mouth, but actually the body begins preparing well in advance. Just the sight, smell, or even the thought of food triggers higher levels of saliva production in your mouth, along with an increase in the movements and acid production of the stomach. That is where terms such as "mouth watering" and "stomach growling" come from. The digestive system is gearing up for what is to come, both chemically and mechanically.

The foods we eat come in a variety of different shapes, sizes, textures, consistencies, and flavors, to say nothing of the actual nutritional value. A glass of milk and a T-bone steak couldn't be more physically different, yet they contain many of the same proteins, fats, and carbohydrates. As a liquid, milk doesn't really require any mechanical digestion, or movement on the part of our body to aid in digestion. Even a newborn can digest mother's milk. But to digest a big chunk of steak, it must be mechanically changed.

Typically we start the process of mechanical digestion by cutting large pieces of solid food into smaller, bite-size pieces. While it is possible to digest a large chunk of food without chewing it, that is very inefficient. Cutting solid foods into smaller pieces greatly improves the effectiveness of the digestive process.

Chewing is an important part of mechanical digestion for several reasons. Our teeth are designed to tear and grind pieces of food into increasingly smaller particles, which can be more easily swallowed. Chewing also mixes the food with saliva, which is produced by several glands inside the mouth. Saliva acts as a lubricant that makes the food easier to swallow, and it also contains some digestive enzymes called amylase. These enzymes begin the process of chemically altering some carbohydrates, even before you swallow them.

There is a lot of truth to what your mother told you: "Slow down and chew your food." We always seem to be in a hurry, and it takes time to chew many foods adequately. In fact, eating too fast, taking large bites, and not chewing adequately are all eating habits associated with obesity.

But mechanical digestion does not stop with chewing. When you swallow, the food passes from the back of your throat down into the stomach through a tube called the esophagus. The stomach is a large pouch that can easily hold a liter or more of food and fluid. It produces a highly concentrated solution of hydrochloric acid, capable of breaking down the structure of even the toughest foods we ingest.

Mechanical digestion in the stomach is not limited to the effects of acid. The stomach acts like a big mixer, mechanically transforming the food into a thick paste. It literally grinds the food using rhythmic contractions of the muscles of the stomach wall, known as peristalsis. This type of "milking" action occurs naturally throughout the GI tract and is how food is propelled along. At the bottom of the stomach there is a muscular valve, called the pylorus, which prevents food from passing out of the stomach until it is about the consistency of oatmeal. The pylorus remains closed as the rhythmic contractions of the stomach muscles turn it into a "mixer." Once the food has been combined with the acid and ground into mush, it is ready to be released by the pylorus into the small intestine, where the remaining chemical processes of digestion take place.

The Liver, Pancreas, and Chemical Digestion

The process of changing complex substances—like a piece of chicken or an apple—into tiny, submicroscopic molecules that can be absorbed into the bloodstream takes more than just chewing, swallowing, and letting the stomach grind for a while. It is really beyond the scope of this book to explain all of the various chemical reactions required to complete the task of digesting a meal. However, the principle to remember is the need for bile and digestive enzymes to break apart large, complex molecules into their smaller component parts.

Most of the things we eat are easily dissolved in water and can be thoroughly mixed in the stomach, but, as we all know, "oil and water don't mix." Even though our food is mixed thoroughly inside the stomach, fatty foods tend to collect as separate oily globs within the otherwise watery fluid as it passes out of the stomach. Before fatty foods can be digested, these oily collections must be broken into tiny particles, or globules. That process is called emulsification, and the key to emulsification of fatty foods is bile. Produced by the liver, bile is added to the food as it passes into the first part of the small intestine, known as the duodenum.

Bile helps to break down large fat globs more or less the same way that soap seems to eliminate grease when you wash the dishes. It breaks down the natural surface that exists between oil and water. The fatty material is converted into tiny droplets, which are more evenly mixed in with other food particles in the surrounding watery fluid.

Getting bile from the liver into the intestine involves a system of tubes, called bile ducts. The gallbladder is a small pouch located under the liver that acts as a temporary storage area for bile. As the stomach fills up with food, a hormone called cholecystokinin is released into the bloodstream. This hormone stimulates the gallbladder to contract, literally squeezing bile out of the gallbladder, through the main bile duct and into the intestine. In this way a large amount of bile can be added to the food precisely when it is needed most.

Unfortunately, the gallbladder is a frequent source of problems, including gallstones. These are actually just crystallized bile, and when they occur they often require the surgical removal of the gallbladder. Since the gallbladder is merely a storage container, removing it does not prevent bile from being added to the food, but the system does not work as efficiently as it normally would. Generally that is not a problem unless you eat a large, fatty meal. Without a gallbladder to add large amounts of bile all at once, some of the fatty material may pass through the intestine without being completely digested. These undigested fats are irritating to the lower intestines, causing diarrhea or abdominal cramping. That is why people who have had their gallbladder removed are generally told to avoid really fatty meals.

The mechanical actions of chewing and the mixing of food with acid inside the stomach, as well as the action of bile on fats, are each important, but the real digestive process occurs on a molecular basis. The chemical changes that break down our food require a group of highly specialized molecules called digestive enzymes. It is these enzymes that make it possible for the food we take into our mouths to make it ultimately into our bloodstream for general distribution throughout the body. For purposes of simplification, there are three main categories of enzymes. Each category is named for the type of material that it helps to digest. Amylase is the enzyme that works on starches and other carbohydrates, converting them into simple sugars. Lipase works on lipids, or fatty substances, breaking them down to fatty acids, cholesterol, and other absorbable fats. Protease breaks complex protein molecules into their building blocks, known as amino acids.

The salivary enzymes were mentioned earlier in the mechanical section, but they are also part of the chemical digestion process. Saliva contains the enzyme amylase, which begins the process of chemically breaking down carbohydrates. The amount of amylase in the saliva is relatively small, especially compared with the amount produced by the pancreas. The majority of amylase and virtually all of the lipase involved with digestion are produced by the pancreas and are added, along with bile from the liver, directly to the food as it passes out of the stomach. If it were not for pancreatic enzymes, we simply could not digest even the most basic foods.

Since both bile from the liver and enzymes from the pancreas are not added to the food until the first part of the small intestine, known as the duodenum, chemical digestion doesn't really begin until the food reaches this point in the alimentary tract. The precise location where pancreas enzymes and bile are added to the food we eat is important, as it pertains to obesity surgery, because a person's anatomy can be surgically altered, greatly affecting the overall digestive process. In other words, by rearranging the digestive system the surgeon can actually change a person's ability to digest and absorb certain foods.

Unlike amylase and lipase, protease enzymes are for the most part produced by the cells that line the inside of the small intestine. These powerful chemicals can quickly turn the protein in a steak into amino acid molecules small enough to be absorbed directly into the bloodstream.

Absorption and Conversion

Once food has been mechanically and chemically broken down into its basic components, the final part of the digestive process involves getting those tiny molecules of simple sugars, fatty acids, amino acids, vitamins, and minerals out of the intestine and into the bloodstream. All this occurs in the small intestine. It is about 18 feet long and about an inch to an inch and a half in diameter. But the lining of the intestine, the actual surface area where the absorption of nutrients occurs, is many times larger than it appears. That is because of the presence of millions of tiny fingerlike projections called villae that blanket the inside of the intestine.

Each villus contains a tiny network of capillaries capable of absorbing molecular nutrients directly into the bloodstream. Larger fatty molecules are absorbed into the villus and then are taken up by a tiny one-way channel called a lacteal, which eventually connects with the bloodstream via the lymphatic system. This process of absorption is very efficient at taking up virtually all available nutrients, in no small part because of the presence of millions of villae, which greatly increase the total available surface area in which nutrients can be absorbed.

Some molecules that are absorbed into the bloodstream, such as ammonia, must be chemically altered before they make their way into the main circulatory system. Otherwise they will cause serious toxic reactions, particularly in the brain. To avoid this situation, all the blood from the intestinal tract first passes through the liver for detoxification. The liver also performs a variety of chemical reactions that change absorbed nutrients into material that is usable by other tissues in the body.

Immediately after eating, the amount of the simple sugar, glucose, present in the bloodstream exceeds the amount needed by the cells. The liver converts much of this simple sugar back into a more complex molecule called glycogen, which is then stored in the liver. As the available glucose in the bloodstream gets used up, the liver can quickly convert these glycogen stores back into glucose for use as a cellular energy source. This system helps to avoid major fluctuations in the availability of glucose during periods between meals. However, if sugar and fat intake consistently exceeds the needs of the body, the glycogen stores continue to build up inside the liver and can lead to what is frequently referred to as a "fatty liver." Over time this can even interfere with the normal functions of the liver.

When the total amount of nutrients taken into the body consistently exceeds the material and energy needs, the body turns the excess into long-term storage in the form of fat. This includes all forms of excess nutrients, including even pure protein. Do not be fooled into thinking that fat comes only from sugar and starchy or fatty foods. Within the liver, chemical reactions occur that can turn excess amino acids into glucose, which is then converted into fat.

The medical term for stored fat is adipose tissue, and it can be found in nearly every part of the body. The exact location and distribution of major fat stores depends on age, gender, genetics, and, of course, how much excess fat there is. Major deposits of adipose tissue can create "apple" and "pear" shaped bodies, round faces, prominent abdomens, and all the other outward appearances we associate with obesity. If the amount of nutrients taken in is less than the body needs, these fat stores can be mobilized, and the contour of the body will change.

It is important to realize that not all adipose tissue occurs in areas of the body that can be easily seen. Fatty deposits also occur around major organs inside the body. These so-called visceral fat deposits, especially those around the heart, can actually interfere with the normal function of the organ.

The bottom line is that a healthy diet is one that meets the needs of the body without consistently exceeding those needs. Excessive intake always leads to excessive stores of fat, and that is likely the reason you are reading this book, right?

Waste Management

Not everything we eat is nutritious. That is true even for those people who claim to eat only healthful foods that are high in nutritional value. Some stuff is just not digestible and therefore passes through the intestine without being absorbed. We often refer to that kind of material as roughage, and a certain amount of it is good for us. Everything we eat moves through the small intestine, and anything that is not absorbed passes into the large intestine for eventual evacuation.

The job of the large intestine, also called the colon, is simply to concentrate the leftover material by absorbing most of the water out of it. This occurs as the waste moves through the 5 or 6 feet of colon and is eventually passed out of the body as feces by way of the anus.

If it weren't for a certain amount of roughage, the waste would end up being very small, creating small and firm stools. To move that type of fecal material along requires the colon to generate pressures that are much higher than normal. Over time those high pressures become the main cause of a common condition known as diverticulitis. So, having some roughage in your diet is clearly a good thing.

Summary

Eating a meal is one of the simplest and most basic of all human activities, but the process of digestion is actually quite complicated. The things we eat must be broken down into their basic molecular components. Then they are absorbed into the body, detoxified, and chemically changed by the liver into building blocks and energy sources the body can use. Any nutrients absorbed through the intestine but not used immediately are stored as fat for future use. Everything that is not absorbed is discharged as waste. Thank goodness the process is automatic.

Now that you've seen the basic components and processes of the digestive system, it's time to take a look at various types of weight-loss surgery, how those modifications work, and what the trade-offs are in terms of risks and benefits.

4

Bariatric Surgery

Past and Present

> *Yet it is equally clear that knowledge of what is*
> *does not open the door directly to what should be.*
> —Albert Einstein, *Ideas and Opinions*

To put it mildly, obesity is a very complex problem, but everyone seems to be looking for a simple solution. I've had a number of people say to me, "Just wire my mouth shut, Doc." Or they'll ask, "Can you just sew up my stomach so I can't eat anything?" Interesting ideas, but as we learned in the last chapter on how the digestive system works, the fact is, you've got to eat. Every human being must have nutrition; it's part of living. It is also inconceivable that one single treatment, even surgery, could successfully change a lifetime of overeating.

Bariatric surgery is a relatively recent addition to modern medicine and is still evolving today. Within the last half-century or so, a number of different operations have been developed specifically to treat overweight patients. Each successive procedure has gone through a number of changes and refinements, trying to balance safety and effectiveness.

The word "bariatrics" comes from the Greek word *baros*, which means "weight." We've all heard meteorologists talk about "barometric pressure," which is basically the weight of the atmosphere on any given area of the earth's surface. In medical terminology, bariatrics is defined as the study and treatment of the problem of excess body weight.

Obesity as a Disease

Before getting into specific weight-loss surgery procedures, there is a major question that has yet to be satisfactorily answered regarding obesity. Is it a condition, or is it a disease? While physicians have always recognized the problem and its harmful effects on their patients' health, until recently it was a widely held opinion that obesity was more of a social disorder than a medical condition. For that reason it has been largely ignored by the mainstream medical community. This belief was supported by the notion that there were no effective treatments.

As the obesity epidemic has continued to spread, however, the problem has come under increasing scientific scrutiny, and several major medical organizations such as the World Heath Organization and the National Institutes of Health have acknowledged obesity as a disease. However, this designation continues to be questioned, especially by the health insurance industry. As it turns out, this is an extremely important debate, given the fact that health insurance policies cover only proven treatments for recognized diseases. Obviously, if obesity becomes universally accepted as a true disease, the health insurance industry's financial exposure is potentially huge.

Over the last several years it has been very interesting to hear patients explain why they are seeking bariatric surgery. More often than not their statements involve improving their health. Sometimes they are even more specific, suggesting that they have been diagnosed with diabetes or high blood pressure and that has made them realize the effect their weight is having on their overall health. What I find most interesting is how frequently patients tell me that the idea of looking into surgery as a treatment for a lifetime of obesity was theirs, not their doctor's. That is in part because the medical profession has had virtually nothing to offer morbidly obese patients other than surgery, and many internists and family physicians do not consider surgery a reasonable option. On the other hand, more acceptable medical treatments are invariably prescribed for conditions that are clearly secondary to obesity. Diabetes, hypertension, sleep apnea, back pain, and knee and hip arthritis are all treated with a pill or other treatments, while their primary cause, obesity, goes virtually unmentioned.

Historically, other widely misunderstood conditions have taken a long time to reach disease status. Among them are many psychiatric problems, such as schizophrenia and bipolar disorder, and neurological conditions such as Alzheimer's disease. Part of the recognition process of these disorders as diseases has been the development of medical treatments, even if the treatments were not very effective.

The absence of any specific medical treatment for obesity, combined with a built-in bias that suggests obesity is actually the result of personal laziness or lack of discipline, creates a setting in which obesity as a disease is still being debated. The outcome of this debate has far-reaching consequences, because obesity has reached epidemic status, and providing surgical treatment would prove extremely costly to insurers. What can't be debated is the devastating effects obesity has on the individual's health. In recent years medical treatments for obesity have been increasing. Let's take a look at these treatments.

Drugs Used to Treat Obesity

While the condition of obesity has been around forever, it wasn't until about 50 years ago that it began to be recognized as a major health risk in the United States. As the problem continued to grow, public demand for a solution also increased. Health clubs that stress the need for exercise became a national phenomenon in the 1970s and continue to be extremely popular today. But for people who are truly morbidly obese, the results of exercise alone have been disappointing, to say the least.

Numerous appetite suppressants and metabolic stimulants have been introduced over the years, including drugs such as Meridia® and Phenteramine®. While these drugs have enjoyed some success in helping those who need to lose a few pounds, they have been disappointing when the problem is morbid obesity. Perhaps the most successful of these drugs was Fen-phen, which was a combination of Fenfluramine® and Phentermine®. Both of these appetite suppressants had been around for many years, but they were not used in combination until the early 1990s. Shortly after Fen-phen was introduced, it was being prescribed by many physicians for their obese patients. In some cases the results were dramatic. Patients swore by Fen-phen because it significantly suppressed their appetite. But in 1997, Fen-phen and another similar drug, Redux®, were taken off the market after being linked to the development of a type of valvular heart disease thought to be life threatening. Unfortunately, no other drugs before or since have yielded the same level of weight loss.

There is another drug, Xenical®, which works in an entirely different way. It binds up ingested fat inside the intestine, preventing it from being absorbed. The idea sounds good, because it seems to indicate that you can eat anything you want and the fat will just go right on through. But again, there are potential nutritional side effects, because certain fatty acids and essential fat-soluble vitamins are also bound up and can not be absorbed into the body. Also, it is important to remember that not all calories come from fat. Absorption of simple sugars, complex carbohydrates, and protein are not affected by Xenical®, so it is still possible to gain weight when taking this medication.

A variety of over-the-counter appetite suppressants and metabolic stimulants have also been touted for their potential to cause weight loss. If only their claims were true, the problem of obesity would simply disappear. The list of medical and semimedical options continues to get longer but with minimal effect on the growing epidemic.

Surgical Treatments

In the 1960s, a few surgeons began experimenting with various operations designed to achieve significant weight loss. These surgeons were generally criticized by the medical community as a whole. Such "experimental" treatments were considered illogical, inappropriate, and dangerous. Despite this criticism, over the last half-century many different surgical procedures have been developed and performed to achieve weight loss. They have ranged from literally wiring the patient's jaws shut, to placing a large balloon inside the stomach to take up space. Liposuction and other plastic surgery procedures that physically remove fat have also been touted as effective means of achieving weight loss. Many of these procedures offer little in the way of success and have been advocated by only a handful of surgeons. Some were not much more than passing novelties and as such do not deserve anything beyond a casual mention.

Other procedures were more widely adopted within the surgical community. These bariatric operations fall into one of two basic categories: restrictive and malabsorptive. Restrictive bariatric operations limit the amount of food that can be eaten, while malabsorptive procedures interfere with the absorption of nutrients by the intestine. Some procedures employ both elements to some degree. Each type of procedure has its own set of benefits as well as its own set of problems.

Jejuno-Ileal Bypass
(also known as the JI Bypass or Intestinal Bypass)

One of the most commonly performed bariatric operations in the 1960s and 1970s was the jejuno-ileal bypass. It was also commonly called the intestinal bypass. The procedure simply shortened the small intestine from its usual length of about 18 feet to only about 4 feet. The concept was to minimize the absorption of food, regardless of how much the individual ate.

The small intestine is composed of three parts: the duodenum, the jejunum, and the ileum. The duodenum is the first part of the small intestine and is about 1 foot long. The second part is called the jejunum and constitutes approximately half of the small intestine. The remainder of the small bowel is called the ileum, which extends from the midway point to the end, where the small bowel empties into the colon.

Each part of the small intestine absorbs different nutrients. Certain things that are absorbed in the jejunum are not absorbed in the ileum, and vice versa. In particular, some vitamins and bile salts are absorbed only in the very last part of the small intestine, called the "terminal" ileum. Armed with this knowledge, when surgeons performed any procedure to shorten the small intestine, they tried to maintain at least part of both the jejunum and the terminal ileum; thus the name of the procedure: jejuno-ileal bypass.

Following JI bypass, patients typically experienced significant and rapid weight loss. Many patients praised this operation as the "cure" for their obesity. However, as time went by, a large number of patients developed serious side effects as a result of this rearrangement of their intestines. Problems included dehydration, kidney stones, uncontrollable diarrhea, anemia, malnutrition, various vitamin deficiencies, and even liver failure. Eventually deaths began to be reported as a result of what came to be known as the JI bypass "short-gut" syndrome.

The increasing frequency and severity of major complications resulting from JI bypass only added to the general perception among physicians and surgeons that obesity was anything but a surgical disease. Those who actually performed bariatric surgery were more or less shunned by the majority of the surgical community. Even so, many of these early pioneers were convinced that the answer to the numerous complications of JI bypass rested solely in their ability to leave behind precisely the right amount of each part of the intestine. For more than a decade arguments raged over the exact number of centimeters of jejunum as well as the length of terminal ileum that should be left behind to cause the desired weight loss while avoiding nutritional complications.

Ultimately, by the end of the 1970s, the JI bypass had fallen completely out of favor and was replaced by somewhat safer procedures, performed on the stomach and designed to simply restrict food intake. Logically these became known as gastric restrictive procedures.

Gastric Restrictive Procedures

In the second half of nineteenth century a German surgeon named Theodor Billroth became widely recognized as the father of gastric surgery. He developed many of the techniques that are still used today for removing parts of the stomach, and reconnecting it to the small intestine. Prior to the mid 1970s there were no medications like the ones we have today, which are capable of suppressing the stomach's ability to produce acid. As a consequence stomach ulcers were a common and often serious problem frequently treated by surgery to remove large parts of the stomach. In those days ulcer operations constituted a major part of virtually every surgeon's practice. These procedures have been performed not only as treatment for ulcer disease but also as treatment for stomach cancer in more or less the same way for over 100 years.

Since the very early years of gastric surgery, it was recognized that after these procedures many patients experienced significant weight loss. In fact, that was considered one of the more serious and undesirable side effects. The stomach normally can hold a quart or more of food and fluid. Naturally, if a significant part of the stomach is removed, or bypassed, it will have a significant impact on the amount of food the individual is able to eat at any given time. For many patients, a smaller stomach created real problems just maintaining adequate nutrition. But for those who were morbidly obese to start with, having a major gastric procedure was just what they needed to lose weight. Ultimately, these experiences led surgeons to begin using these operations solely for the purpose of achieving weight loss.

In the 1960s, surgical stapling devices became available and were a major technological innovation, especially for stomach operations. They made these operations quicker and easier because they divided the stomach and at the same time sealed the edges closed with staples instead of sutures. This made cutting out portions of the stomach faster than the more traditional techniques, and offered better control of bleeding and potential postoperative infections. Eventually staplers were designed simply to seal tissues like the stomach closed, without actually dividing them. Surgeons soon learned to modify these devices to perform a simple weight-loss procedure, which became known as "gastric stapling." A few of the staples could be removed from the middle of the stapler so that when placed across the upper part of the stomach, the device would essentially create two compartments with a small opening between them.

The amount of food the patient could eat was restricted, because the upper part of the stomach was purposefully made small so that it would fill up with only a very small meal. Eventually, food makes its way out through the small opening into the rest of the stomach to be digested. This procedure enjoyed considerable acceptance among bariatric surgeons because it appeared to work fairly well and offered much lower risk than the JI bypass.

Gastric stapling does cause considerable weight loss, but the results simply don't last. The problem is that the opening between the two parts of the stomach tends to stretch out over time. This allows patients to eat larger and larger meals because the food moves quickly from the upper compartment into the lower compartment. As a result, most patients tend to put back the weight they lost within just a few years. In an attempt to address this problem, the vertical banded gastroplasty was developed.

Vertical Banded Gastroplasty

Eventually, the gastric stapling procedure was modified to help eliminate the problem of stretching of the opening between the two parts of the stomach. The staple line was oriented more up and down rather than across the stomach, and the opening between the two parts of the stomach was encircled with a ring that would not allow it to stretch. The ring was made of steel wire that was wrapped in silicone to prevent the wire from cutting through the stomach wall. Once this permanent band was in place, it maintained the size of the opening between the two parts of the stomach. This procedure became known as the vertical banded gastroplasty, or VBG. For much of the 1980s it was the most commonly performed bariatric procedure.

Many of those who performed the VBG once again believed they had found "the answer" to the problem of morbid obesity. Patients were losing weight rapidly, and the risk seemed to be relatively low. But on closer inspection the long-term results were like those of previous operations—less than optimal. Although the banded opening could not stretch, the upper stomach pouch often became stretched. This dilated stomach allowed patients to eat more, and they gained much of their weight back. Likewise, staple failure was a frequent problem because patients would overeat, and the pressure inside the upper stomach pouch would eventually cause some of the staples to come loose. Loose staples meant that new paths were created for food to pass through to the lower stomach compartment. The end result was that patients were able to eat more, with predictable results. There were also other concerns with procedures like stomach stapling and VBG.

Nutritional Concerns

Despite the frequent long-term failures with both stomach stapling and VBG, these procedures continued to be performed, largely because they were much safer than JI bypass. Both procedures maintained all of the normal absorption of nutrients in the small intestine. As long as the patient ate a balanced diet, the problems of malnutrition, vitamin deficiencies, and anemia could be avoided. This sounds simple enough, but it requires a great deal of effort to undo years of dietary indiscretion and overindulgence and develop better nutritional awareness.

Likewise, patients with small upper stomach compartments and intact staples often found it hard to follow the postoperative eating guidelines, which included eating smaller meals and thoroughly chewing all foods.

Since the procedures were so restrictive, many patients switched over to eating things that would go through easily. Liquids go down quite easily, so eating ice cream and drinking milkshakes or other high-calorie liquids was common. The problem is that most of these foods are high in calories yet lack adequate nutritional balance. They are typically short on protein and high in carbohydrates and fat. After a few years, many patients reported they had gained back much of the weight, and were also experiencing hair loss and muscle wasting.

Gastric Bypass (or Roux-en-Y)

From the late 1970s and into the 1980s, vertical banded gastroplasty was the darling of the bariatric surgical community. However, as late failures began to mount up, an operation began to be used that was based more on the surgical resections that Billroth had pioneered a century before. The Roux-en-Y gastric bypass that is commonly used today to treat morbid obesity was a modification of what is known as a subtotal gastrectomy, a procedure in which most of the stomach is removed. This operation was one that was commonly used in the treatment of ulcer disease for the previous four or five decades. The difference between the subtotal gastrectomy and a gastric bypass lies in the fact that in the latter the bulk of the stomach is not actually removed; it is merely bypassed. The word "Roux-en-Y" is a surgical term used to describe how the small intestine is connected to the small stomach pouch.

To perform a Roux-en-Y gastric bypass, the surgeon first divides the stomach, creating a very small stomach pouch just below the esophagus. The intestine is then divided near the beginning of the jejunum. The lower end of the divided intestine is brought up to the small stomach pouch and sutured or stapled to it. This allows food to pass directly into the intestine, bypassing the rest of the stomach. To complete the procedure the surgeon needs to reconnect the upper end of the divided intestine back into the small intestine downstream.

Following the Roux-en-Y reconstruction of the upper intestinal tract, the stomach is not the only area being bypassed. As we learned in the last chapter, bile and pancreas enzymes are both added to the intestine in the duodenum. Since food is also being diverted around the duodenum, these important chemicals are not available to help digest fats and carbohydrates until after the food gets down to the point where the two parts of the intestine are rejoined.

One of the biggest arguments among bariatric surgeons involves just exactly how long the segment of intestine should be that extends from the stomach down to where the small intestine is reconnected. This is commonly called the small bowel limb, or the bypass limb. The pancreatic enzymes and bile enter back into the main stream of the intestine at this point, and only then can they begin to digest the food. So it would only seem logical that the longer the small bowel limb, the shorter the intestine that remains available to absorb nutrients. But the fact is that unless the limb is extremely long, it has very little impact on digestion. We have much more intestine than we actually need, and unless the length is extremely short, as in the JI bypass, absorption of nutrients is usually not significantly impaired.

When performing a Roux-en-Y gastric bypass, the size of the stomach pouch is very important. If it is too big, the patient is able to eat too much and will fail to lose weight. If it is too small, the patient may have difficulty maintaining adequate nutrition. But as was the case with the VBG, it is important to recognize that the stomach is quite stretchable, and with time the pouch is likely to stretch out. So, in general it is a good idea to start out too small rather than too big.

The size of the opening made between the stomach and the small intestine is also very important. If the surgeon makes it too big, the food just goes right through, and the patient never gets a sense of satisfaction. As with the stomach stapling procedure, it is not uncommon for this opening to stretch over time, leading to late weight gain.

Another complication can occur as a result of this new connection between the stomach and intestine. It is fairly common for the opening to become very narrow. This is due to excess scar tissue or acute inflammation caused by ulcerations at the site of connection. The latter usually occurs within a few weeks after the surgery, while narrowing caused by scar tissue may not show up for years. In both cases the opening may be dilated, but if the narrowed opening cannot be stretched enough it may require reoperation to enlarge it.

Despite these and other problems, the Roux-en-Y gastric bypass is still the most commonly performed technique used in bariatric surgery today. There have been a number of modifications, including one in which the stomach is simply stapled closed and not actually divided, followed by connection of a Roux-en-Y limb up to the upper gastric segment. As you might expect, the problem with this option is once again the failure of staples, allowing food to pass through.

Another modification avoids constructing the Roux-en-Y altogether. A loop of the intestine is simply brought up to the stomach and connected to the pouch. This procedure frequently leads to a variety of problems including ulcers and chronic abdominal pain as pressure builds up inside the intestinal loop. Generally speaking, these procedures are being performed by only a few surgeons and are not considered mainstream bariatric procedures.

Kathy's Story

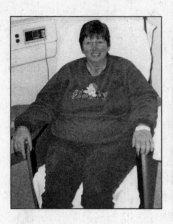 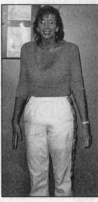

(Left) Kathy, pre-op, 373 pounds.

(Right) Kathy, nineteen months post-op, 145 pounds.

I had every major health problem. I was diabetic, had a hiatal hernia, high cholesterol, high blood pressure, sleep apnea, arthritis in my knees and elbows, and more. I took 15 pills a day to survive, and I couldn't even walk up steps. I started at 373 pounds, and I'm 5 feet, 8 inches tall. My doctor told me to get 150 pounds off or I wouldn't see my next birthday. I was in tears. I was about to have my first grandchild, and I didn't know if I would even get to hold her.

I did Weight Watchers®, TOPS, the cabbage diet, and more. I'd say there wasn't a diet I wasn't familiar with. I got to the point where I'd go on a diet, lose 20 pounds, and no one could even tell. Of course, then I'd put back on double.

I opted for the gastric bypass. I didn't know about the band, but looking back I probably wouldn't have chosen it anyway. I looked on the Internet into gastric bypass and everyone was having complications down the line, so everything I read was against it. And when I told people, all my family and friends were against it, including my husband and my doctor. But the way I looked at it, I was going to die anyway, so what did I have to lose? If I had it, at least I could say I was trying.

I found out, I couldn't just go out and have bypass surgery. A doctor had to recommend it for my insurance to pay. So I took my husband, who was having a headache problem and doesn't speak much English, to a doctor who speaks fluent Spanish. While we were there I asked the doctor about bypass surgery, and he said he thought it was a good idea. He said he'd seen remarkable things with the bypass, and I'd be a good candidate. My husband was better about it then. The doctor wrote me a full-page recommendation about how obesity affected my health. He asked me questions, but I could tell he knew the story. I told him how I couldn't fit into a booth in a restaurant or an airplane seat, couldn't ride in an amusement park ride, and all the usual stuff.

I went to three different doctors' seminars, so I felt I knew exactly what was going to happen. But the barrier was still insurance. We submitted to insurance and they denied it. We resubmitted and they said okay, but I found out they were going to stop paying for it as of the end of the year. I had surgery on December 21, just 10 days before the cutoff date. I went home December 22 and went back to work the next day. I work at the phone company, so I didn't really take any time off. I had to work Christmas Eve and Christmas Day, too, because I would have lost all my holiday pay if I hadn't.

After surgery I stuck to the liquid diet, then went to pureed foods. I never had much of an appetite after the surgery. I eat to stay healthy, not because I'm hungry. I eat because I have to eat to keep my bones healthy, and to keep my hair. From the very day I came home from the hospital, I started exercising. I started walking around the block a couple of times, and worked up to 2 miles, then up to 10 miles a day. On my lunch hour, I work out at Curves®. I also started riding a bicycle instead of walking, and I kept going to Curves®.

Nineteen months out from my surgery, I weigh 145 pounds. I lost 25 pounds the first week after I had my surgery. I lost 10 to 15 pounds a week after that. I probably leveled off about a month or so ago. I don't actually have much hanging skin except on the inside of my thighs. Some plastic surgeons say you cannot get rid of the loose skin without surgery, but that wasn't true for me. I worked out and firmed up a lot.

I'm at 145 now, and the charts say I'm underweight and should be between 150 and 177. My cholesterol and everything is perfect. My blood pressure is down, and my blood sugar is great. I had follow-ups with my surgeon every three months. But he said I don't have to go back to him unless I fall under 150 pounds and that happened, so I did see him again. But he didn't have much to say about my weight. I did meet with a dietician a couple of times before the surgery and in the hospital. And I have a number for her, but I haven't talked with her since I was in the hospital.

I have experienced dumping syndrome a couple of times. If you do it once you don't want to do it again. What I ate ran right through me, and I didn't have any way to stop it. I don't eat sweets like chocolate. I also have had several episodes when I felt like I was having a heart attack. It felt like something was stuck in my chest and I couldn't get it to go up or down. I've thrown up a couple of times since my surgery, and it's more like foam that comes out. It hurts to throw up.

I've always been outgoing, but I notice people treat me differently. I feel a lot better about everything now. I know other people have had a lot of trouble with the bypass, but I think the difference between me and someone else is I followed the exercise program exactly the right way.

Biliopancreatic Diversion

There is a variation of the Roux-en-Y gastric bypass called the biliopancreatic diversion (BPD), which significantly shortens the functional intestine. In this procedure the small bowel limb is reconnected down near the end of the ileum. This operation combines both the restriction of a small pouch and the malabsorption effects of a short intestine. The weight loss following such procedures is often dramatic, but not surprisingly, patients have some of the same complications that were seen with the JI bypass.

Another similar modification of this operation is the biliopancreatic diversion with duodenal switch (BPD-DS). In this procedure the size of the stomach is reduced by performing what is called a sleeve gastrectomy, which converts the stomach into a long tube. The remaining portion of the stomach pouch is actually removed, the rationale being that many of the hormones that cause hunger are produced in this large stomach pouch. The duodenum is divided and the outlet of the stomach is connected to the small intestine, allowing the food to bypass the bile and digestive enzymes from the pancreas. The remaining part of the small intestine containing this "biliopancreatic" fluid, which is required to allow digestion of fats and carbohydrates, is reconnected well downstream, near the end of the ileum.

Both of these procedures are usually reserved for patients who are extremely heavy, with a body mass index (BMI) over 80; a category often referred to as "super obese." As you might imagine these extremely complex operations, performed on extremely obese patients, carry a significant risk of a variety of complications.

In an effort to reduce the risk, some surgeons have elected to perform the BPD-DS as two separate operations. The first procedure is the sleeve gastrectomy. That is then followed several months later with the rearrangement of the small intestine. Many patients tend to lose a substantial amount of weight following the creation of a gastric sleeve, and this can significantly reduce the risk of their second procedure. Some surgeons have recently started using the gastric sleeve procedure alone as a purely restrictive weight-loss operation for patients who are not good candidates for other procedures, or who want to avoid the higher-risk gastric bypass. The early results with the gastric sleeve are promising, but for those patients in the super obese category, it is generally recommended they proceed with the rearrangement of the small intestine procedure six months to a year after the gastric sleeve procedure.

Results of Roux-en-Y Gastric Bypass

The Roux-en-Y gastric bypass procedure and its variations are often called the "gold standard" for bariatric procedures because the weight loss is predictable and rapid. When done properly, weight loss after a gastric bypass can be 5, 6, or even as much as 10 pounds a week.

Rapid weight loss is really appealing to a patient who wants a "quick fix," even though he or she has spent a lifetime becoming overweight. Once patients make up their minds that they want to do something, they tend to believe that "faster" is "better." That's not necessarily true, and, in fact, very rapid weight loss is often accompanied by serious nutritional problems. What amounts to a crash diet can lead to inadequate intake of protein, certain vitamins, and essential fatty acids, as well as important minerals and other nutrients. This can constitute a big problem, especially if allowed to continue over an extended period of time.

One of the inherent problems with any procedure that bypasses the bulk of the stomach is a form of vitamin deficiency that shows up as anemia. Vitamin B-12 plays an important roll in the process of making red blood cells, which carry oxygen to the body. B-12 is also very important to ensure normal nerve function. A critical process actually occurs within the stomach that influences the absorption of Vitamin B-12. When the bulk of the stomach is bypassed, patients tend to develop anemia because they have trouble absorbing this essential vitamin even if they are taking in iron-rich foods or iron supplements. Anybody who has a gastric bypass needs to be getting B-12 regularly, to avoid anemia as well as serious neurological problems.

The most serious potential problems associated with gastric bypass are related to the fact that when the stomach is divided, it requires reconnection of some type to the intestinal tract. This new connection needs to heal without leaking, and even in the most skilled hands there is always the possibility of a leak. If the liquid contents within the stomach leak out into the abdominal cavity, it will likely result in a serious and sometimes life-threatening infection, especially if not diagnosed right away.

Among the other complications of the various bypass and stapling surgeries is the development of an incisional hernia. If the wound doesn't heal completely the edges of the muscle can separate, creating a defect in the abdominal wall called an incisional hernia. This can occur in any patient, but for those with diabetes or who smoke cigarettes the risk is quite high because both conditions interfere with wound healing. Overall, about 20 percent of patients who undergo bariatric procedures using open abdominal incisions end up with hernias, which ultimately require additional surgery to repair.

As bariatric surgery became a more acceptable treatment option, more and more surgeons began to perform these procedures. Many have been forced to reconsider that decision after experiencing one or more serious operative complications as well as rising liability insurance premiums. Today bariatric surgery still bears some of the stigma of being too risky. Some have also suggested that it is being performed by surgeons more concerned about money than the health and well-being of the patient. While there are probably some surgeons who fall into that category, for the most part bariatric surgeons are extremely conscientious and make every effort to provide their patients with safe and effective options for this difficult disease.

Laparoscopic Surgery

In the 1980s the first laparoscopic gallbladder operation was performed by the German surgeon Eric Muhe. Gynecologists had used this technique for many years to perform tubal ligations to sterilize women and even removed ovaries without making a large abdominal incision. The first laparoscopic gallbladder operation performed in the United States was performed by J. Barry McKernan in 1988. While others soon followed, this technique was initially criticized by most surgeons, much like bariatric surgery.

Eventually more surgeons and, most important, the public in general realized that laparoscopic surgery offered many benefits including smaller incisions, less pain, and faster recovery. This minimally invasive technique rapidly evolved, and within a few years it was used to take out appendices, repair hernias, and even remove spleens and parts of the colon. It became apparent that with the proper set of technical skills virtually any intra-abdominal procedure could be performed using the laparoscopic technique. Eventually a few experienced surgeons even began performing gastric bypasses using the laparoscopic technique, thus avoiding most of the complications related to the big, open incision.

At about the same time the National Institutes of Health (NIH), a part of the U.S. Department of Health and Human Services and the primary federal agency for conducting and supporting medical research, published a consensus paper on obesity. That paper essentially defined morbid obesity as a serious medical problem associated with diabetes, high blood pressure, and many other significant health threats. They went on to suggest that surgery had been shown to be the only truly effective long-term treatment for the problem of morbid obesity. The paper said that only 5 percent of people who go on a diet lose their weight and keep it off, while a high percentage of people who have surgery to lose weight are successful at keeping their weight off.

The combination of this rising awareness about obesity as a serious health risk and the ability to perform laparoscopic gastric bypass created a major increase in the number of these procedures by the mid-1990s. A significant factor in the rise of laparoscopic gastric bypass was its obvious marketability. Laparoscopy obviously provides major advantages to the patient in terms of lowered pain, increased comfort, and shortened recovery time. These advantages were enthusiastically promoted, and the public was quick to recognize the benefits.

Unfortunately, the majority of the surgical community was still in the early phase of developing laparoscopic skills when this procedure first started becoming popular. By the late 1990s, a number of surgeons started offering these very complicated procedures to the public, and some had not yet developed the necessary laparoscopic skills or experience to perform these procedures. Complications—especially leaks from the point where the small intestine and the stomach are sewn together—are more difficult to recognize when working in the laparoscopic environment, so many procedures that were started as laparoscopic operations were ultimately converted to open operations. Even as late as 2005, the majority of gastric bypass procedures were still being performed through large open incisions despite all of the hype and marketing of the laparoscopic technique.

Without question, the laparoscopic gastric bypass has become the procedure of choice in most bariatric surgical practices, but many patients remain cautious about the risks and the permanence of rearranging the anatomy of the stomach. In recent years, laparoscopic surgery has given rise to another option that is rapidly challenging gastric bypass because of its relative safety and effectiveness. The adjustable gastric band (AGB) is a procedure ideally suited to laparoscopic surgical techniques.

The Problem with Any Surgical "Solution"

Unfortunately, many patients approach weight-loss surgery of any kind with the attitude that they are now "fixed." They have this opinion because in most surgical cases for other problems, the procedure does in fact provide the solution. Bariatric surgery and the AGB are the exceptions.

With any bariatric operation, there has always been a need for careful follow-up and nutritional counseling. Regrettably, in the past some surgeons offered their patients very little other than periodic examinations during the first few months after surgery. In part this was because they really couldn't do anything surgically to assist the patient once the procedure was over. All they could offer was a referral to a dietitian or nutritionist for counseling.

What has further compounded the problem is that not many dietitians are experienced in dealing with the special needs of bariatric patients. Often these professionals are not particularly supportive of the patient's decision to have the procedure in the first place. Some dietitians put the blame for failure back on the patient's poor food choices, their lack of exercise, or on the operation itself.

A fair number of bariatric surgical patients have simply been sent back to their internist or family physician to manage their various medical problems. Physicians who are unfamiliar with these procedures often criticize the patient's decision to have bariatric surgery as illogical or inappropriate. That is unfortunate, since many of these patients are already living with the stigma of "having to resort to surgery." The perception of such treatments by some in the medical community is that they are only necessary for people who have "character defects" such as a lack of willpower or laziness. (Does this sound familiar?)

Over the last several years, bariatric surgeons have gradually begun to recognize the true importance of careful long-term follow-up after weight-loss surgery to help patients deal with the psychological and dietary aspects of obesity surgery. The critical importance of appropriate exercise and lifestyle changes also began to receive more emphasis in the overall management of obesity.

Having said this, it is very important to point out from the outset that AGB is more of a behavior-modification tool than it is a true bariatric procedure in the traditional sense. The keys to success include more than just the laparoscopic procedure to place the band. Regular follow-up with appropriate adjustments to the band, support from other band patients, and nutritional and psychological support and counseling are all components to help bring about the variety of lifestyle changes for success with the AGB. The remainder of this book is dedicated to this procedure and the important nonsurgical elements that make up a comprehensive AGB program.

The Adjustable Gastric Band (AGB) Is Not Gastric Bypass

5

How the AGB Functions

Any sufficiently advanced technology
is indistinguishable from magic.
—Arthur C. Clarke, *The Lost Worlds of 2001*

In the last chapter we looked at the various types of bariatric surgery and determined that while the adjustable gastric band (AGB) is weight-loss surgery, it doesn't really fall into the category of traditional bariatric surgery. The AGB is a tool, and the purpose of this chapter is to offer details about how it is placed and how it functions.

Overview of the AGB's Function

The basic idea behind the AGB is really quite simple. The band acts like a tourniquet around the upper part of the stomach, limiting the amount of food you can eat. It artificially separates the stomach into a small upper pouch and a much larger lower pouch. The lower pouch receives food only as fast as the band will allow. (Please see the figure on the following page.)

The upper pouch fills up quickly and empties slowly. Restriction of the intake of food is created without the risk of stapling, diverting, or rearranging the stomach or any part of the digestive tract. The fact that the band doesn't require rearrangement of the digestive system explains why the AGB is the safest surgical option currently available for the management of obesity.

Controlling the amount of food the stomach pouch can hold is only part of the way the AGB works to promote weight loss. Perhaps the most remarkable effect of the band is its ability to reduce hunger. Anyone who has ever been on

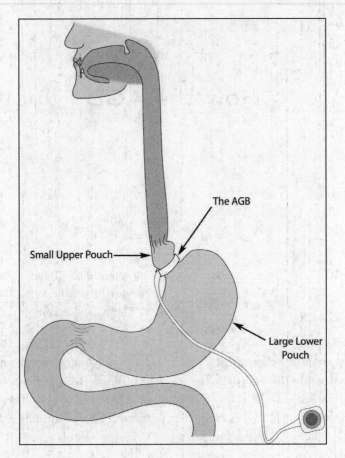

Like an adjustable tourniquet around the stomach,
the band limits food consumption.

a diet knows that hunger is the main reason for failure. It takes only a small amount of food to fill the space above the band completely, yet patients report that the feeling of fullness is the same as if they'd eaten a sizable meal. Food tends to stay in the upper pouch for several hours after a meal, creating a sense of satiety.

Further, patients who have a band often say that they are simply not hungry, even when they haven't eaten anything. The physiologic reasons for this seemingly miraculous effect are not completely understood. However, it seems likely that the presence of any food or fluid within the upper pouch stimulates nerve impulses or hormones to be released from the stomach that shut off the hunger center in the brain. As a result, some people enjoy the absence of hunger for prolonged periods of time.

The key to making the band work is creating just the right amount of restriction. When it is appropriately adjusted, the band promotes weight loss, but at the same time it will allow adequate amounts of food and water to pass through into the rest of the digestive tract. If the band is too loose, it will not offer enough restriction to be effective. If it is too tight, it will severely block the flow of food and fluids through the stomach, leading to malnutrition or even acute dehydration.

When the band is properly adjusted, the opening between the two parts of the stomach is fairly narrow, like an hourglass. To achieve the proper amount of restriction, the band is inflated by injecting saline solution into a small reservoir that is placed under the skin and attached to the band by a length of tubing. The band can also be loosened by removing some or all of the saline. While this sounds pretty easy, properly adjusting the band can be quite challenging, and an entire chapter of this book is dedicated to the process.

Surgical Placement of the AGB

The operation to place the AGB is almost always performed using a technique known as operative laparoscopy. Sometimes this type of surgery is referred to as minimally invasive because there is no large incision as is common in traditional surgery.

The advantages of laparoscopy include less pain, faster recovery, and fewer noticeable scars. It is particularly beneficial for obese patients, since they are known to have higher surgical risks. Patients are subjected to less trauma, so they require less pain medication. They are up walking around more quickly and can resume normal activities right away.

During laparoscopic surgery a small tube, called a cannula, is placed into the abdominal cavity through the skin and muscular wall. The cavity is then inflated with carbon dioxide gas, similar to blowing up a balloon. The pressure of the gas creates space for the surgeon to work between the internal organs and the wall of the abdomen.

A long, thin telescope, called a laparoscope, is attached to a high-intensity light source and a miniature video camera. The camera is connected to a high-resolution video monitor so that when the laparoscope is inserted into the abdomen, it offers the surgeon an extraordinary view of the internal organs.

Additional cannulas are inserted through the abdominal wall as conduits for specialized instruments to be used by the surgeon to perform the operation. The surgeon and entire team are able to watch every move on video monitors.

To expose the area of the upper stomach requires the liver to be physically lifted off the stomach. The liver is often quite large and somewhat immobile in very obese patients. This can prove to be a major obstacle in working around the upper part of the stomach. In extreme cases a large "fatty liver" can make it nearly impossible to perform the procedure safely. To avoid this situation and make the procedure safer and easier, my patients are placed on a preoperative low-fat, low-carbohydrate diet for three weeks. (I present the details of the diet in Chapter 8: What to Expect before Surgery on pages 99–100.) This pre-op diet can pay big dividends, because the liver usually shrinks dramatically in just a short time.

During the surgery, an initial dissection of the upper stomach area is performed prior to placing the band. An experienced surgeon can usually accomplish this in just a few minutes, but the process can take considerably longer depending on how much fat is present around the lower esophagus and upper stomach. As a rule, the dissection tends to be more difficult in men than it is in women. Obese men have more fat around the stomach and other areas inside the abdomen than do obese women, who tend to carry more of their fat under the skin. When the band is in the right spot, it will create an upper stomach pouch that holds only a couple of ounces of food.

To be effective, the AGB must be placed around the stomach in the proper location. If it is placed too high, the pouch will be too small to hold enough food to allow for adequate nutrition. It is actually possible to place the band around the esophagus, which can lead to problems, including difficulty swallowing, blockage of the swallowing tube, or even injury to the esophagus.

If the band is placed too low, the pouch will be too big to be effective for weight loss. This makes the band ineffective for helping the patient lose weight. Also, if the band is too low, heartburn is a common symptom.

There are two bands that are most popular, primarily because they were the first two to be offered to the public, but there are sure to be many variations as the band gains popularity. The most popular band is 10 centimeters in circumference and holds about 4 cubic centimeters of saline. Another popular band is 11 centimeters and holds 10 cubic centimeters of saline.

Most of the time the smaller-size band can be placed around the stomach and the surrounding fat without any difficulty. However, if too much fatty tissue is included inside the band, it can cause early obstruction, which means that the band is so tight not even fluids can pass through. This problem can be avoided by removing some of the fat before the band is placed. But removing fat may be quite difficult and runs the risk of injuring the stomach. A better choice is to use a larger band, one designed specifically to avoid the possibility of early obstruction.

Once the appropriate band is selected, the surgeon first inflates it with saline to ensure that it doesn't leak. It is then deflated and inserted into the ab-

domen through one of the cannulas. An instrument is passed behind the stomach to pull the band tubing around. Then the tubing is threaded through an
opening in the end of the band and is gradually pulled through until a locking
mechanism snaps the band closed around the stomach. During this step there
is a slight risk of injury to the stomach or other organs in the area.

The surgical risk depends in large part on the amount of fat around the
stomach and the laparoscopic experience of the surgeon. An injury to the back
wall of the stomach can be difficult to detect because the surgeon can't really
see back there. If a perforation occurs in that area it can have disastrous consequences, especially if it is not immediately recognized. The spillage of stomach
contents into the abdomen will nearly always lead to a major, life-threatening
infection. Fortunately this is uncommon with the AGB, in comparison with
other procedures such as gastric bypass.

An unrecognized hiatal hernia can also increase the possibility of problems
while placing the band. (If part of the stomach pushes up through the muscles
of the diaphragm, that is called a hiatal hernia.) This situation is actually quite
common and is frequently associated with heartburn. If a small hiatal hernia is
found, it should be repaired before the band placement can continue.
However, if the hernia is larger than an inch and a half, the band may not be an
appropriate choice. This situation is associated with a higher incidence of problems after surgery, including displacement of the band and possible recurrence
of the hernia. In patients with symptoms of heartburn or chest pain or regurgitation of food prior to surgery, it is a good idea to have some type of testing to
rule out a large hiatal hernia before deciding on the band.

Putting a band around the stomach is a bit like placing a ring around a balloon filled with water. The stomach is a very flexible, saclike structure, and over
time it can change shape dramatically. If the AGB is not secured in some way, it
will likely slide up or down as the stomach shifts around. To secure the band
where it needs to remain, the surgeon pulls a portion of the stomach wall up
over the band and sutures it above the band. The idea is to trap the band within
a tunnel created by the stomach wall. This holds the band in much the same
way as a belt loop holds a belt. A small percentage of bands escape this tunnel
and start to slip up, or more often down, on the stomach. That is called band
slippage, and this subject will be covered in detail later in this book.

Once the band is secured into place, the end of the band tubing is brought
out of the abdominal cavity through one of the cannula openings. The tubing is
then tunneled under the skin and attached to a reservoir, called the "port." The
port is made of hard plastic, with a titanium steel bottom. The front of the port
is specially designed with a silicon rubber plug, which can be penetrated with a

specialized needle passed through the skin. This allows saline solution to be injected to adjust the tightness of the band. The silicon plug reseals as the specially designed needle is removed.

Most often the port is placed on the upper left side of the abdomen, but it can be situated almost anywhere on the abdominal wall. It only has to be accessible with a needle placed through the skin. Once the port is in place, it is covered by a layer of fat. The thicker the fatty layer the more difficult the port is to feel through the skin. For this reason, some surgeons elect to put the port up on the breastbone, where the fatty layer is generally thinner. While this location makes the port easier to feel and access with a needle, the result can be a visible swelling and a bump between the breasts. This will become even more obvious as the patient loses weight. For this reason, most surgeons prefer to place the port on the side of the abdomen.

Once the port has been sutured to the muscle, each of the small skin incisions is closed with dissolvable sutures. Small dressings are used to cover each incision site prior to the patient's leaving the operating room. Although this marks the end of the operation, for the patient it is only the beginning: the patient now has a new tool to help in the fight against obesity.

The AGB from a Surgeon's Viewpoint

As a surgeon, I am accustomed to taking direct treatment actions to correct any number of problems. Many physicians are drawn to a career as a surgeon because ailments with surgical treatment as an option—such as appendicitis and hernia—are "fixable."

The surgeon's job typically involves making the diagnosis, explaining the procedure to the patient, and performing the operation. For many acute illnesses or conditions, the surgeon acts like a healthcare "firefighter." Once the patient has recovered from surgery (that is, the fire is out), the surgeon's work is done.

The surgeon's job stands in sharp contrast to many chronic medical conditions, which require long-term management. Obesity is just such a long-term problem, even when it is treated with an operation. Our modern society is constantly being advised that a "quick-fix" exists for virtually everything from bad breath and wrinkled skin to heartburn and insomnia. We obviously want just such a solution for obesity. We witness numerous promises of rapid weight loss and find it difficult to believe differently.

When I first started treating obese patients with the AGB, it was natural for me to think of the band operation the same way I have other surgical procedures. While I certainly understood that there were other issues that would need to be addressed, I hoped the procedure alone would lead to successful weight loss. That was clearly a false assumption. As I watched patients struggle with making the lifestyle changes I recommended, it became obvious what they really needed was a program to back up the procedure.

Getting our patients to understand that the AGB is not a cure-all for their weight problems has been the greatest challenge my staff and I face. Many patients come to us with the preconceived notion that getting a band means that they will never have to worry about their weight again. This is simply not true. The AGB is a tool. The surgical procedure is merely the installation of that tool, not an automatic weight-loss operation.

Dan's Story

I'd always been fat. My top weight was 355. I was 340 in my before photo, and 323 when I got banded in 2003. Now, four years later, I don't think of the change in my body just in terms of weight loss, but in changes in my life. My pants used to be a size 56 and are now a size 38 or 40. My shirts were 3X or 4X, and are now XL. I shop in regular stores, and not just in the "fat guys" store. I can also fit in restaurant booths, exercise easily, and do a whole host of other activities (even though I just had my sixty-fourth birthday) that just weren't possible when I had another 140 pounds on my body.

I work for a university library as the network information coordinator, and I lead the SmartBandsters, a Yahoo group aimed at helping people who are banded. I've seen thousands of people post their questions and concerns. One of the things I find is so many people, no matter what kind of weight-loss surgery they have, think they'll be magically cured. That's not so. The best analogy I have for life with the band is peeling away layers of an onion. There's always another layer underneath, especially if someone has been eating for psychological reasons.

I'm a recovering alcoholic and so is my wife. We've both been married before. One of the pluses for me working a 12-step program is that I've already dealt with a lot of my issues. I've found, being banded, that compulsive eating is like drinking. Things that tend to put the average drinker on to alcohol are described by the acronym HALT—hungry, angry, lonely, or tired. I know to watch myself if I'm in one of those four states of mind. Food is always there. And food is harder to handle because it's socially okay to eat, while drinking and drugs are not as socially acceptable.

There's a saying in AA, one scotch is too many and 100 is not enough. It's the same for me with various foods. Frito Lay had a commercial that said, "Betcha can't eat just one." No kidding. I know I can't have just one potato chip or one M&M. But with alcohol or drugs, I can simply avoid them. I can't stop eating. I have to fight that devil three or more times a day. What makes it more complicated is I'm eating in the presence of other people who can deal with food in more of a "normal" way. They can have just one and be okay.

While the band restricts my eating, one of the things the band will not stop me from is "grazing." If I'm eating three or four small meals a day, that'll work. But if I'm at a buffet the whole day and I just keep nibbling for several hours, then I'm going to eat several days' worth of food. So I work to avoid situations in which I can graze all day.

I'd say there are biological issues with weight, too. For example, some of us have issues with our brain chemistry. Obesity is not caused by a single issue. It is so multifaceted that you've got to deal not only with the physical but also with the rest.

One thing people don't realize is that it's possible with the band to gain the weight back. I believe that's more common with the bypass than the band, because the band gives you more time to modify your behavior. And the band is adjustable, while the bypass isn't. If a person is counting to a considerable extent on the restriction that comes with the bypass, that could be a problem, because the odds are they're going to lose the restriction over time.

I think it's smart for people to be in a band support group beforehand. However, many surgeons who perform band surgery also do gastric bypass. In a situation like that, some practices try to put all the patients in the same support group. I think that's a mistake. Bypass people lose so quickly at first that it can be discouraging to someone with a band who is going to lose more slowly, at the rate of a pound or two a week. And there are also other issues unique to band people that might not get addressed or are passed over in a mixed group.

One of the issues unique to band people is what some call productive burping, or PB-ing. It's more like baby spit-up, since it's coming from above your band. You can call it anything you want, but I found I had this problem until I learned to chew well. The standard is to chew 20 times, while putting down the fork between bites. Many people are used to shoveling food into their mouths in a hurry, such as when they're driving or eating in front of the television. Before I was banded, I was watching a football game and at half-time I realized I'd eaten the entire big bag of chips. I thought the dog had gotten into the chips, but then I remembered we didn't have a dog anymore. I've found mindful eating works better. I think about what I'm eating and pay attention with each bite to see whether I'm full or not.

After I got a band, I also realized that I had never experienced physical hunger, because I was eating all the time. Further, I'd never learned to discern the difference between physical and emotional hunger. Or knowing hunger from thirst. I've found that some people eat when they're thirsty. Learning those differences is important to band people, and it takes time.

I have modified some of the band "rules" in my own life. For example, I drink water, right up until I start a meal. Then I put the water glass away and tell the waiter or waitress I don't need a refill. I figure the water will run right through the pouch and won't wash food through if it is taken in first. But I stop drinking as soon as I start eating.

I have other tricks I use. For example, when they bring the meal in a restaurant, I ask them to bring the carry-out box at the same time they bring the food. Before I start eating, I divide my meal into a smaller portion and put the rest into the carry-out box. When I wasn't banded, I never took a carry-out box home from a restaurant. My parents grew up in the Depression, and we were poor. So we were taught to clean our plate, and I didn't leave the table until I was done—even if it meant eating eggplant, which I hated. That type of training put me in a position to clean my plate. So now I just make sure I don't have too much to eat when I start.

What I also see a lot is that band people don't want to exercise. I think exercise is another important change you have to make. Even when I weighed 355, I lifted weights, but I didn't jog like I do now.

Band people would be smart to decide beforehand if they want to tell people they're banded or not, and who they want to tell. Once you tell, you can't un-tell. One of my sisters is head of medical records in a big hospital, and when I let her know I wanted to get a band, she reamed me. I told her, "You know me, I do research for a living. I've researched the band very carefully." Then I gave her some sources and suggested we talk again after she had checked it out. She called back in a few days and apologized.

I've only had three fills. I just haven't needed more. What I notice is that band people always want to talk about the size of the band and the amount of the fill. I think it's irrelevant, so I just don't talk about it. Fills are like Goldilocks and the Three Bears: it's either too big, too little, or just right. And the amount of the fill that works depends on the individual.

I've also had plastic surgery, a tummy tuck, to handle the excess skin around my middle because it was bothering me. I considered doing more, since I have excess skin on my arms, chest area, and inner thighs. But I asked my wife and she doesn't care. Since it doesn't bother me either, I decided not to have any more plastic surgery.

Changing behavior is the big thing. I see it a lot working with band patients online. There are always some who will keep spitting up every meal because they insist on doing things the way they've always done them. If they continue, they can dilate the pouch, erode the band, and all sorts of other things can happen. There are always a few who have their band taken out, almost always for behavioral reasons. And a few where the band and their stomach just don't get along. I've heard a lot of people who had reflux before the band don't have it anymore after they're banded, and others who never did have reflux experience it after they have a band. It seems there's never just one totally simple answer.

I don't see myself as a missionary for the band, but I am an educator. If I can help people by educating them, I'm happy to do so.

Is the Adjustable Gastric Band
Really Bariatric Surgery?

I am often asked if the AGB is bariatric surgery. As I pointed out in the previous chapter, all bariatric operations are classified as restrictive or malabsorptive, or in some cases, both. A restrictive procedure physically limits the amount of food you can eat, while a malabsorptive operation reduces the amount of food that can be absorbed in the process of digestion.

The adjustable gastric band is classified as a purely restrictive procedure. However, what makes it different from all other bariatric operations is the fact that the amount of restriction can be adjusted to meet the individual patient's needs. Most important, the adjustments can be made without the need for any additional surgery.

Adjusting the band ensures that every patient gets a custom fit. As a patient's circumstances change over time, the tightness of the AGB can be altered to meet those changing needs, such as pregnancy or other medical conditions. This is a truly unique feature, which makes the AGB the most versatile surgical option available for managing obesity.

Unlike typical bariatric operations, the AGB does not cause weight loss by itself. I commonly refer to the AGB as a pair of weight-loss "crutches." For someone with a broken leg, crutches can allow them to be mobile. However, the crutches don't walk by themselves. They are simply the tools the patient uses to accomplish the goal of ambulation. It is not enough that the individual wants to walk and buys crutches. They must also supply the energy to use the tool in order to walk.

Like the crutches, the AGB is a tool used by obese patients to gain control of their weight. The band provides guidance, encourages better eating habits, and strongly discourages overeating. It is a training tool designed to help the patient accomplish the weight-loss results they have been unable to achieve through willpower alone.

The results will depend in large part on how willing the patient is to change the behaviors that caused their obesity. If they are committed to making real changes in their eating habits and lifestyle, the band will provide the discipline. Through personal commitment, along with the support of a skilled team, remarkable results can be obtained.

But, as with any training process, the keys to success include both the motivation of the student and the quality of the instruction. Once properly installed and adjusted, the AGB can be used to help patients control how much food is taken in. In this sense, and in my opinion, the AGB is not like traditional bariatric surgical procedures. It is instead a very effective tool for a lifestyle change designed to interrupt the obesity cycle.

Breaking the Cycle of Failure
G. Dick Miller, Psychologist

There is a cycle of failure characterized by the punishment paradigm, which is this: "Pay attention only to negative behavior, and if positive behavior exhibits itself, ignore it." That type of thinking doesn't work. What works is instant feedback and positive reinforcement. In order for change to take place, it's necessary for the reinforcement to be stronger than the punishment. In other words, the brain must have a good emotional experience.

There's not much about eating right in the short-term that produces a good emotional experience for the brain. For example, if an overweight person eats well for a week, no one will say they're doing a great job. And it's entirely possible that after seven days of excellent food choices, the overweight person may not lose any weight. This amounts to the punishment paradigm, ignoring positive behavior.

But with the band, individuals know immediately they're eating less, and they feel satisfied, not hungry. Having a band is like the first two weeks of taking diet pills. It's easier to avoid abusing yourself with food when you're not driven by excessive hunger, when you feel satisfied. Of course, the body adjusts to diet pills after a short time, but the band doesn't have that limitation.

Further, the band is monitoring consistently, patiently, 24 hours a day, seven days a week. After a while, it's just easier to stop trying to get around it.

It's important to note that people who lost weight with the band didn't do so because the band changed their eating habits. The person changed. Patients can and sometimes do fight the band until they learn to change their thinking through positive reinforcement. What's great about the band is that it works despite rotten self-talk and self-depreciating language on the part of the patient. Whether anyone notices or not, many banded people are not hungry, know they ate less, know they feel better, and know they're transforming. No one is making them change; they're changing, and they know it. And that knowledge revolutionizes the way they feel about themselves.

I like the band because it's so clean—it provides consistent feedback and constant reinforcement. But, as in the use of any tool, patients must be *honest* so they get the correct fills and so nonworking thinking can be addressed by the professional qualified to help.

With all the components of a comprehensive band program—the doctor to make adjustments to the band, the dietitian to act as an eating guide, the exercise therapist to provide coaching and encouragement to exercise, and a psychologist to help patients change their thinking—the band becomes the number one tool to create an environment in which it is much easier for patients to treat themselves well and make smart choices. Overall, the band is *the* tool to help weight-loss patients break the cycle of failure.

Using the AGB as a Behavior Modification Tool

The ability of the AGB to restrict the amount of food, along with the absence of hunger, makes it sound like a magical solution to the problem of obesity. However, it is not quite that easy.

It has often been said that the definition of insanity is doing the same thing over and over again and expecting a different result. That is particularly applicable when we look at all of the various things people do in an attempt to lose weight. The fact is that nothing works unless it is accompanied by a true change in behavior and a corresponding change in lifestyle. The key to successful weight loss with the AGB lies in how each individual patient uses it as a tool to effect those changes.

The AGB is not a diet, at least not in the usual sense of the word. When the band is properly adjusted, you should be able to eat virtually any food—you just can't eat as much. Making good food choices becomes crucial to ensuring proper nutrition. But weight-loss success with the AGB is ultimately linked more to the way you eat than what you eat.

Willpower alone is rarely sufficient to overcome the strong human tendency to resume comfortable behavior patterns developed over many years. To effect a major change generally requires both positive feedback from the new behavior, and a significant penalty for continuing the old behavior.

The AGB provides continuous restriction, offering immediate negative feedback for undesirable eating behavior. If you eat too fast, take a bite that is too big, or attempt to overeat, the band will let you know. It acts like an unseen "drill sergeant" providing continuous discipline. That is why we have affectionately come to refer to our Comprehensive Weight Management Program as "Dietary Boot Camp."

If you don't eat slowly and chew all foods thoroughly, the band will make you miserable. A bite that is too large or not adequately chewed will feel like it is hung up. The trapped food causes the esophagus to contract vigorously in an attempt to push the bite through the narrow opening created by the band.

This spastic contraction is very uncomfortable and is usually felt in the chest. The pain often radiates into the back or up into the neck. It is usually accompanied by the production of a large amount of foamy mucus, which quickly builds up in the esophagus above the blockage. Salivation can also increase in the mouth as the body attempts to provide lubrication. Some band patients call this "sliming."

Eventually, the mucus, along with some or all of the recently swallowed food, will come back up. This is not really vomiting, and doesn't contain much, if any, digestive acid. It is more of a spontaneous regurgitation. Some patients refer to this spitting up as a "productive burp."

The same symptoms will occur if you eat too fast. Even small bites will be a problem if they aren't chewed thoroughly. With the AGB, it becomes critical to take your time while eating. I recommend that you get in the habit of setting your fork or spoon down on the table after each bite. This conscious effort serves as a reminder to slow down. If you don't, the "drill sergeant" will remind you.

Checklist: Tips to Successful AGB Eating

✓ Take your time to eat.
✓ Take small bites, about the size of the tip of your index finger.
✓ Chew each bite thoroughly.
✓ Put your utensil down between bites while you chew.

Virtually every patient who has a band has experienced the pain associated with eating too fast or taking bites that are too large. Most have also endured the embarrassment of having to excuse themselves from the table as the bite they just swallowed comes back up. While unpleasant, for many this is precisely the motivation they need to change their old eating habits.

Summary

The adjustable gastric band is a weight-loss tool. First, it must be properly placed. Then it must be appropriately adjusted. Finally, it requires continuous monitoring and support as new eating behaviors lead to a change in lifestyle.

In addition, there is a clear distinction between the AGB and procedures that we typically classify as bariatric surgery. With this tool, weight loss is not automatic, but occurs only with significant behavior modifications and lifestyle changes. In the next two chapters we will explore who is a suitable candidate for the AGB and why—as well as what kind of support programs are needed to achieve long-term success.

6

Who Is a Candidate
for the AGB?

People grow through experience if they meet life
honestly and courageously. This is how character is built.
—Eleanor Roosevelt, *My Day*

When we look back on our lives each of us can identify certain major milestones. Some were the result of events that we couldn't control. Others were things that we specifically caused to happen by virtue of our own actions. Making major decisions of this nature takes courage, whether they be buying a home, changing jobs, or deciding to do something definitive about chronic obesity.

Every patient I see has a different story to tell about how they came to their decision to get an AGB. However, what is common to each story is an underlying awareness that they've tried everything and nothing seems to work. Ultimately, the majority of my patients tell me that their decision was in fact one of those life-altering milestones.

Coming to a Crossroads—
Treating Obesity as a Disease

For many people the decision to have surgery to help them lose weight comes only after extensive research. For others it may be the result of having personally observed the success of a close friend or family member. Regardless of what triggers that decision, it makes sense only if you have come to the realization that you aren't able get control over your weight by yourself. This is tough, because we invariably feel like a failure whenever we have to admit we can't do something on our own.

Prospective patients frequently start out trying to explain to me all the reasons why they haven't been successful losing weight on their own. Before they get too far into their list I stop them and ask, "Do you think you could treat your own heart attack?" Obesity is a disease, and like any other disease it requires professional treatment. Once you learn to view it as such and recognize that being involved in a weight-management program is in fact a medical treatment designed to control that disease, your success will come much easier. The true crossroads isn't the decision to get a band; it's the decision to change the way you look at your obesity.

The Minimum Criteria

While your actual weight in pounds and your specific BMI are important, I think it is of greater importance to look at individuals and how their weight affects their health, both now and in the future. But everyone is obsessed with numbers, so what follows are "the numbers."

Back in Chapter 1 we talked about Body Mass Index (BMI) and how it is used to create the categories of obesity. A BMI of 25 to 30 kg/m² is classified as "overweight." A BMI of 30 to 40 kg/m² is classified as "obese." A BMI above 40 kg/m² is classified as "morbidly obese," and one over 80 kg/m² falls into the "super obese" category. Anyone can calculate their own BMI using the formula BMI = body weight in kilograms divided by height in meters squared. Generally it is easier to determine your BMI using a chart like the one provided in the Resources section of this book (page 261).

Most surgeons agree that patients should meet some minimum criteria before even considering bariatric surgery. This is not something that should be done for someone who needs to lose just 20 or 30 pounds. A number of years ago, the American Society of Bariatric Surgeons (ASBS) developed some general guidelines for its members to use when evaluating patients for weight-loss surgery. Under those guidelines, for a patient to be considered for any type of bariatric surgery, including the AGB, they should have a BMI greater than 40 kg/m², or a BMI greater than 35 kg/m² with at least one significant medical co-morbidity, such as Type 2 diabetes, hypertension, sleep apnea, major arthritic changes, or gastroesophageal reflux disease. The patient's obesity should also be a chronic problem, generally of five years' duration or longer, and during that time the patient should have made a reasonable effort to lose weight through dieting and exercise.

Checklist: General Criteria for Weight-loss Surgery Patients

(Established by the American Society of Bariatric Surgeons)

✓ BMI greater than 40 without a medical co-morbidity
✓ BMI greater than 35 with a medical co-morbidity*
✓ Obesity chronic for five years or longer
✓ Reasonable efforts made to lose weight through dieting and exercise

Clearly, insurance coverage is a huge issue for most prospective patients. But the fact is that each and every policy is different, creating an extraordinarily challenging set of problems. However, virtually all policies that offer coverage for bariatric surgery have adopted the ASBS guidelines as criteria, which must be met before the patient can be approved for any weight-loss procedure. These guidelines were never meant as absolute rules for performing bariatric surgery, but, with the dramatic increase in demand, the insurance industry has elected to adopt them as rigid criteria for paying weight-loss surgery claims. That can be a major source of conflict, because the "criteria" are not always followed in determining whether a claim is paid. And, as I eluded to, many policies have specific language in them that excludes coverage for any bariatric surgery. It is also important to realize that insurance coverage for bariatric surgery, and the AGB in particular, can be added to the list of excluded procedures by the insurer without notification at the annual renewal of the policy. Such exclusions for bariatric surgery take effect immediately, so just because a policy covered the band operation one year, doesn't mean it will cover it the next.

While it is relatively easy to measure your BMI, the presence of co-morbidities can be and often is disputed by insurance companies. Despite the presence of "written criteria," arguments frequently arise when attempting to define the "medical necessity" for bariatric surgery. Even after getting letters from physicians and documenting medical conditions, many patients are also required to document their weight-loss efforts. As you might expect, those efforts are then subject to interpretation. Some policies require that specific dieting efforts be under the direct guidance and supervision of a physician, but even then the level of supervision can come into question.

When patients find out that their insurance doesn't cover the cost of bariatric surgery, or the band in particular, the most common response I hear is, "Don't

---

*Significant co-morbidities include Type 2 diabetes, hypertension, sleep apnea, major arthritic changes, or gastroesophageal reflux disease.

they understand that I am going to cost them less in the future when I no longer need medications for diabetes and high blood pressure?" While this sounds like a reasonable argument, the fact is that insurance companies are not in the business of investing in your future health. The economic benefits of weight loss are obvious, but they are realized over a number of years. The insurance company has no assurance that you will remain insured by them beyond the current contract year, so they have little incentive to provide coverage based on future savings.

Another insurance issue is somewhat unique to the AGB. Following the procedure, the band must be adjusted, often several times over a period of months. These adjustments are not part of the procedure, and therefore the insurer may not pay for adjustments even if the operation was covered. Likewise, most policies don't even recognize a comprehensive weight-management program, but instead place all of the emphases on the surgery. This inappropriately discounts the other elements critical to the patient's success.

Without question, insurance coverage makes it possible for some people to access healthcare who might not otherwise have the means to pay for it. But at the same time there are many others who are denied bariatric care through this system. The system has evolved to the point where many, if not most, people perceive that healthcare is available only through their insurance. Therefore, if they are denied coverage for obesity surgery they feel they have no other choice. To address this problem, many surgical practices offer a number of financing options for those without insurance coverage. That allows patients to choose for themselves how they wish to deal with this lifelong condition.

The Initial Evaluation

Many surgical programs offer free seminars for prospective patients as a means of providing information in an efficient manner. These seminars can range anywhere from a 20-minute presentation by a nurse or other staff member to a two-hour comprehensive explanation by the surgeon and his or her entire staff. While the seminar can be quite informative, it is not designed to provide individual recommendations. If the seminar is followed by an on-the-spot attempt to get you signed up for surgery, you may want to consider looking elsewhere. The decision to change your life by getting an AGB is one that is very personal and should be made only after careful consideration. Don't let anyone pressure you into making this important decision on the spur of the moment.

It may be a good idea to go to more than one seminar, just to see for yourself what the differences are in the various programs. Once you have made up your mind to move ahead, you will need to make an initial appointment with the surgeon. During this initial appointment the surgeon or a staff member will take a detailed look at your particular situation and let you know about their screening process for prospective patients.

Different programs have different processes for screening prospective patients prior to approving them for surgery. Sometimes this screening includes insurance preapproval before an appointment is even made to see the doctor or a member of the staff. Personally, I believe that excludes many patients who not only would benefit from the program but who also might well be inclined to find a way to obtain financing despite being denied insurance coverage.

At a minimum, each patient should be evaluated by the surgeon to determine whether an AGB is an appropriate option. Subsequent visits with a clinical psychologist and a registered dietitian should also be considered mandatory as part of the presurgical assessment process. Having an exercise physiologist perform an initial exercise tolerance test and a series of body measurements is also a routine part of many programs.

The Surgical Assessment

The first assessment should be by the surgeon. During your initial visit he or she will gather all the necessary medical information, which allows them to provide you with appropriate medical advice regarding the band. They will likely have you fill out a medical information form similar to ones other doctors use. However, for patients with the diagnosis of morbid obesity there are several areas of the medical history that deserve special emphasis. Problems such as diabetes, high blood pressure, heart problems, respiratory problems, sleep apnea, liver disease, or gastric reflux are among the most common conditions associated with obesity. Any one of those conditions can significantly influence your overall risks and benefits in terms of the AGB. Even if you have written down everything on the information form, be sure to make a point of telling the surgeon about these problems yourself. Don't assume, if he or she doesn't bring it up, that it isn't important.

Checklist: Conditions You Would Be Wise to Bring Up When Talking to Your Surgeon about the AGB

(Hint: Don't assume that, because you wrote them on the patient questionnaire, your surgeon knows about these conditions.)

- ✓ Diabetes
- ✓ High blood pressure
- ✓ Heart problems

✓ Respiratory problems
✓ Sleep apnea
✓ Liver disease
✓ Gastric reflux or gastroesophageal reflux disease (GERD)
✓ Hiatal hernia

Potential Road Blocks

There are a number of conditions that can have a direct bearing on AGB surgery. One of the most common is gastroesophageal reflux disease, or GERD. This condition involves the abnormal movement of stomach contents, usually acid, up into the esophagus, causing heartburn, chest pain, regurgitation of food, and other related symptoms. Many of my patients have been on medications for years to reduce the amount of acid produced by the stomach. Not surprisingly, they have also been told repeatedly that losing weight would improve their reflux. Some patients are actually referred for the AGB for weight loss because their reflux has become unmanageable. While the AGB can offer significant relief from GERD symptoms, it is important to recognize that reflux can also be associated with a hiatal hernia, a medical condition involving the stomach and the diaphragm.

The diaphragm is a broad, flat muscle that separates the chest cavity from the abdominal cavity. There is a natural opening in the diaphragm, called the esophageal hiatus, which allows the esophagus to pass through it before emptying into the stomach. The natural resting pressure in the abdomen is significantly greater than the pressure that exists in the chest. The negative pressure in the chest is what allows us to breathe air into our lungs. By contrast, the pressure in the abdomen is positive. In obese patients, their excess weight presses down on the abdomen, further increasing the pressure gradient between the chest and abdomen. That is part of the reason why many overweight people experience shortness of breath.

Over time, the pressure in the abdomen can stretch the hiatal opening in the diaphragm, pushing the stomach through this enlarged opening and up into the chest. This condition is known as hiatal hernia. Since the band is designed to be placed around the top of the stomach, a significant hiatal hernia creates a potential problem because the band needs to be on the abdominal side of the diaphragm to work properly. A small hiatal hernia can usually be repaired at the time the AGB is placed, but for patients with a hiatal hernia larger than a couple of inches in size, the band is generally not a good choice.

For anyone with a history of hiatal hernia, or significant reflux symptoms, it is important to document the presence and size of the hernia. The easiest way to make this determination is with an upper GI X-ray series. The patient is asked to swallow a liquid solution containing barium that shows up on an X-ray. This test will generally demonstrate whether there is a hiatal hernia, its location, and its approximate size. The presence of a hiatal hernia can also be determined using an endoscopic examination of the esophagus and stomach. A flexible, lighted tube is passed through the mouth, down the esophagus, and into the stomach. During this examination the location of the junction between the esophagus and stomach, as well as the position of the diaphragm, is evaluated.

An unsuspected hiatal hernia that is not identified until the time of surgery can create a real problem for the surgeon. While repairing a small hernia as part of a band procedure can be done, it requires more dissection and may also increase the surgical risk. There is also a possibility that later on the hernia repair could come loose and allow the stomach and the band to slip up above the diaphragm and into the chest. It could even result in the surgeon's having to abort the band procedure altogether. So it is far better to know about a hiatal hernia beforehand. If there is any question about the presence of a hiatal hernia, the surgeon will likely order either an upper GI X-ray or an endoscopy before recommending the band. You will certainly want to discuss your situation with the surgeon before deciding whether the band is right for you.

Another medical condition that is common in obese patients is gallbladder disease. If you have known gallstones or have been diagnosed with gallbladder disease, the surgeon is likely to recommend your gallbladder be removed at the same time you have your band operation. That decision will be based on confirmation of gallbladder problems, which will require a gallbladder sonogram or a gallbladder function test called an HIDA scan. It is usually not a problem to combine the elective removal of the gallbladder with the AGB procedure, but if the gallbladder is acutely inflamed or infected, it is generally better to remove it during a separate procedure rather than risking infection of the band.

Chronic conditions that involve the stomach or intestinal tract may also influence whether you are a candidate for the AGB. A diagnosis of inflammatory bowel disease, also known as Crohn's disease, can influence the surgeon's decision regarding whether a band is an appropriate choice for you. Likewise, chronic liver disease, especially when complicated by cirrhosis and dilated veins in the esophagus, known as esophageal varicies, will certainly influence the surgeon's judgment regarding the AGB.

Checklist: These Conditions May Need to Be Addressed Before You Have AGB Surgery

✓ A hiatal hernia (even if you haven't been diagnosed with one, the presence of gastric reflux or gastroesophageal reflux disease is a symptom, and you should be checked for this condition prior to band surgery)
✓ Gallbladder disease
✓ Crohn's disease
✓ Chronic liver disease
✓ Hepatic cirrhosis and dilated veins in the esophagus, known as esophageal varicies.

If after your initial assessment the surgeon tells you that he or she doesn't think the band is a good choice, you may want to get another opinion. If you get the same recommendation from a second surgeon, then you should probably heed that advice, even if you ultimately find someone willing to do the AGB surgery.

During your evaluation by the surgeon, he or she will also explain in detail how the procedure is performed. The surgeon should also go over the potential complications and problems that can occur both during and after the procedure. Sometimes patients are so excited about the prospect of getting a band and starting to lose weight that they fail to pay attention to the surgeon's discussion about the procedure, the downside, or the risks. It's important to pay attention to these explanations and know precisely what you're getting into.

During the surgical assessment your surgeon should also help you establish some realistic expectations about where you are likely to end up and how quickly you'll get there. Virtually every patient has seen the "before and after" photos of individuals who have been extremely successful with the band. You will even see some in this book. In many instances it is those images and the success stories that convinced patients to pursue getting a band for themselves. Obviously, the procedure can be, and is, marketed using those particular patients because they illustrate the optimal results. Not everyone, however, achieves optimal results. So before you assume anything, you should get an idea what the surgeon considers average results. It is important to understand what constitutes poor results as well, and what produces poor results.

In the next chapter we'll discuss how optimal results are related to a comprehensive program offering dietary, exercise, and psychological support in addition to the band. However, it is your willingness and commitment to participate in such a program that will determine just how successful you are. Patients who avail themselves of all aspects of the program will typically lose between 50 and 75 percent of their excess body weight and keep it off. In other words, if you are 100 pounds overweight, you should realistically anticipate losing between 50 and 75 pounds over a period of 12 to 24 months, at the rate of 1 to 2 pounds a week. If you are 150 pounds overweight, the loss should be more like 75 to 115 pounds at the same rate over the same period. Remember, these are average results; some people do better, others not as well.

I have had many patients look at these numbers and suggest that they can and will do much better. In some cases they do. However, the realities are that (1) people who have been overweight for many years are generally unable ever to achieve their ideal body weight, and (2) the objective of the AGB or any weight-loss program is to return the individual to a healthier weight that they can maintain long term. For most patients the loss of at least half of their excess weight represents a significant improvement in their overall health. That is not to say everyone is always satisfied with that result, and perhaps they shouldn't be. The important thing is to establish a realistic target and understand that it is normal to lose between 1 and 2 pounds per week.

You owe it to yourself to be fully informed about all aspects of the surgery. This includes the qualifications of the surgeon, the experience of the anesthesiologist, the capability of facility and support staff, as well as the risks of the procedure and the anticipated results. These are all part of the Comprehensive Weight Management Program, and the time to find out these things is before you proceed.

Once you have been told you are a potential candidate for the AGB, the next steps involve assessments by the other members of the team. Ideally you should be evaluated and advised by a psychologist and a licensed and registered dietitian, along with an exercise physiologist. The purpose of these assessments is to ensure your success by outlining all aspects of the program. Likewise, it will help you to avoid spending time and effort on the AGB if it clearly isn't likely to work for you.

While all of these assessments may make you feel as if you are being placed under a microscope, they also offer you an important opportunity to assess the team that you will be working with in the months and even years to come. Since you are going to be meeting with these people over and over again, you need to feel comfortable with them and believe that they hold your interests paramount. You may want to ask them some questions about their goals and expectations for you, as well as for other patients. It is important that everyone is "on the same page of the program" before getting started.

The Road to Success
Is a Change in Thinking

G. Dick Miller, Psychologist

I see the band as a beginning, a start. A lot of people will get a band, but the ones who succeed will be the ones who change their thinking. These patients move away from the concept that someone is going to do something to "fix" them. They adopt an internal locus of control instead of looking outward.

Many band patients have been out of control for some time, and not only with their weight. Their social and emotional lives have been out of control, too. I see it when I walk into a store. If I'm waiting for a clerk and an obese person is also waiting, I'll get the attention. It's clear to me, when I watch the way heavy people are treated, that they are perceived as being less-than. And it's my opinion that those perceptions lead to an attitude on the part of a heavy person of waiting for someone to give them something that will make them okay.

The successful band person is not waiting for someone or something outside them to change their situation, or give them permission to be all right with themselves. They take responsibility for developing new habits physically, emotionally, and socially. Those who adopt a "wait and see" attitude are on their way to sabotaging themselves. This isn't gallbladder surgery. You cannot just wait for your body to heal and then go about your life the way you did before surgery. It's an ongoing process that begins and centers around change.

And band patients are not the only ones facing a change in their belief system. This requires an adjustment on the part of the surgeon, too, whose training is in cutting and "fixing" the problem once and for all. Many people are waiting for the surgeon to fix them, and the surgeons get angry—sometimes at the patient—if they can't. The gastric bypass fits this "quick fix" description. The band is gradual, which is much safer, but not quick. And it requires ongoing interaction between the medical staff and the patient for adjustments.

My experience is that many people want to believe the hype—that they can just have surgery and it will all be taken care of. But long term it will be the person's belief systems that determine their emotional well-being. "As a man thinketh, so is he," not as the band "worketh or not worketh." A lot of people will get a band, but some will change the way they think. These patients will recognize the band is a tool, but the real victory, the road to success, is in changing their thought process.

The Psychological Assessment

For some, the thought of having a face-to-face meeting with a psychologist can be more frightening than the surgery. "Is this guy going to find out that I really am a little crazy? What if I don't answer all the questions right? Does that mean I won't be a candidate for the surgery?" Nearly everyone has the same concerns, and they are almost always unfounded.

The reason for the psychological evaluation is to help determine the best way to help you achieve success. It is very evident that obesity is closely tied to how we perceive ourselves and our surroundings. There are certainly some causes of obesity that have their very roots in our psyche, and conversely, the presence of obesity often has profound effects on our psychological well-being. The objective of the psychological assessment is to determine within reasonable probability whether you are appropriately motivated and capable of making the behavioral changes needed to be successful. The only way to answer these questions is through an assessment by a trained psychologist.

The evaluation is typically in the form of a personal interview, during which you will be asked a number of questions that will probe into who you are and what motivates you to do what you do. Despite what you may think, there are no trick questions. If you simply answer all of the questions as honestly as possible you will sail through without any trouble. The objective is to find out who you are, not who you think you are or who you would like to be. Psychologists are taught to spot incomplete answers, half-truths, and nontruths, so there is no point in trying to tell them what you think they want to hear. Even if you are successful in disguising your true self, the only person that is potentially harmed is you.

Many psychologist use a written test in addition to a personal interview to determine more precisely the personality traits of the patient. This is still somewhat of an inexact science, but there are some clear patterns of thought and basic beliefs that can be accurately identified through this type of evaluation. While a lot of information can be obtained through testing, the first question that the psychologist is trying to answer is this: Does the individual have sufficient personal insight to accept the fact that their past behavior is what led to their weight problem? If so, do they recognize the need to change their behavior patterns and are they capable of making the necessary changes?

These sound like pretty simple questions, right? Unfortunately, there is no single test or series of questions that can ensure an accurate assessment. In large part that is because many people tend to be less than honest with themselves when it comes to evaluating their own behavior. Getting the most accurate answers often means asking questions in a variety of ways, so don't be surprised if it seems like the questions are repetitive. The objective is to get as clear a psychological picture as possible in an effort to determine whether the adjustable gastric band program is likely to yield the best results for you.

What We Look for in Psychological Testing of AGB Patients
Steven Greer, Ph.D.

When I was brought in initially to run psychological testing on potential band patients for Dr. Sewell, our only source for information was Scandinavian healthcare data. One thing we didn't take into account is how different those systems are. There's no one in Scandinavia who isn't eligible for coverage, although people may have an extremely long wait for care. As a consequence, the Scandinavians used their experience to predict who would fail with the band.

We were warned about certain problems to watch out for, such as severe mental illness, major depression, compulsive people, drug or alcohol dependency, and less self-directed persons. Oddly enough, they said nothing about eating disorders.

So we got a "cannon" of a testing instrument, the MMPI–2, a test that takes on the average an hour and a half to complete, in order to screen for a wide array of psychological problems. We wanted to be very careful about screening.

What we didn't take into account was that in Scandinavia, people aren't paying for any part of their band treatment, so the doctors get absolutely anyone and everyone. We, on the other hand, had to charge several hundred dollars for the testing, which is usually not covered by insurance. What we found is that we didn't see the types of psychological disorders the Scandinavians were describing.

We were given numbers that one out of six people would fail our psychological screening. But what we found was that only 3 percent of the first 100 people we tested ended up having any of the problems we were screening for. People who are seriously depressed or addicted knew it, and they weren't about to pay several hundred dollars to be tested just to be turned down. So, inadvertently, we developed our own screening.

A full 50 percent of the patients coming in to be tested didn't have insurance that covered bariatric surgery. And what we know from other research on self-pay medical patients is that people who pay a significant amount for any kind of medical procedure tend to do better than people who pay nothing. The literature suggests that people are more motivated and more involved when they have a significant financial investment. That's what we were seeing consistently: highly motivated, sophisticated people.

We also know that people who have a religious or spiritual faith, who feel they have an internal source of strength and health, do better in any health category, from cancer to dealing with death. And that also came out in the testing.

The bottom line was that we were seeing hardly any of the things we were warned about. And it came out that some of the things, such as major depression, weren't as much of an issue with the band as we'd been told. Later research in Australia among people who were given a band even though they suffered from major depression, showed they did fine. The depressed people lagged behind others a little in their weight loss, but they didn't show up significantly different than people who weren't depressed.

We were still concerned. One of our biggest concerns was alcoholism and eating disorders, both of which we identified as big league problems for potential patients because those issues put the band at risk. Damage to the esophagus can be a result of either of those addictive disorders, but is especially likely with an eating disorder. With the band, we want people to avoid vomiting because that can throw the band out of place and create problems such as band slippage and erosion, most of which have to be corrected surgically by either repositioning or removing the band.

After the first couple of years, we realized that we didn't need such a comprehensive psychological test. So we switched to tests that take 15 to 20 minutes to complete, including how patients manage their health and a very basic profile of distress.

What we found is that the vast majority of patients who had a weight problem serious enough for them to consider band surgery fell into two categories. One group had a high degree of sociability and gregariousness. They are outgoing and engaging. Since a lot of socializing is done around food, that made sense. These people generally feel confident, some were a little overconfident, and most were independent. The combination of sociability and overconfidence tends to lend itself toward being overweight. These people tend to over-ride their own internal controls because they feel they can take life by the horns and fix things later. They're the kinds of people who will overeat now, thinking they'll eat less either later in the day or maybe on another day.

The second group were very rule-governed, responsible people who want to do all the right things. These people tend to hide their emotions from themselves and from others, are overcontrolled, and sacrifice their own personal interests for those around them. We often refer to these folks as "pleasers." Of this group, the majority were women by nearly three to one. This kind of personality makes for a lot of quiet, "subterranean" needs that food is a handy way to satisfy.

So the majority of what we see in our psychological testing is two personality groups: one group is self-indulgent, the kind of people who think they'll fix it later. And the other has unmet needs and uses food as a substitute for basic gratification that is missing.

We have certainly seen some minor depression, discouragement, demoralization, and restriction of activity caused by the limitations overweight people have. We've often heard complaints to go with these symptoms, such as they couldn't climb three flights of stairs, couldn't play with their kids or grandkids, and couldn't fit very well into an airplane seat. But we almost never saw severe psychotic issues.

What we have found is that attention deficit hyperactivity disorder (ADHD) is a problem for someone who has a band. ADHD is an impulse control problem, and untreated it can potentially lead to problems adjusting to the band.

Bulimia is another issue that we were concerned about. Bulimia is almost always accompanied by a history of sexual abuse, and statistically one out of every eight women has experienced significant, recurrent sexual abuse. If someone is bingeing and purging a couple of times a week and trying to hide it from others, or if they have ADHD, those difficulties need to be dealt with before they actually get a band.

Another thing we looked for is noncompliant personality types, who are very independent and very autonomous. Those are characteristics that tend to lead to overeating to begin with, but these people can also be medically noncompliant, meaning that they have a tendency to be unwilling to submit themselves to medical authority or follow a program. Self-indulgent people tend to give themselves permission not to follow the guidelines put in place by a medical authority, such as their doctor. So we hope to identify these tendencies so that we can provide extra support. These types tend to hit a bump in the road and not make progress for several months to a year. When that happens, the medical staff can find it very frustrating if they're not prepared to handle someone in this position.

So what we have found in psychological testing of potential band patients is different from what we were warned about by Scandinavian data, perhaps because our healthcare system is different. What we now look for are issues that relate to either poor impulse control, such as ADHD, or addictions, such as alcoholism or bulimia. And when we find evidence of these conditions, which hasn't been often, we encourage the patient to seek treatment for those issues before attempting band surgery.

Checklist: Problem Areas We Look for in Psychological Testing with Potential Band Patients.

- ✓ Untreated ADHD
- ✓ Alcoholism
- ✓ Bulimia
- ✓ Severe emotional disturbance.

Checklist: Psychological Factors
that Are Helpful in Living with a Band.

- ✓ Some significant financial commitment toward the band procedure. Research shows that patients having a degree of financial responsibility do better in any medical procedure, and the band is no exception.
- ✓ Religious or spiritual faith. Again, research shows that people who hold these beliefs tend to do better in terms of their health, especially when facing challenging medical situations.
- ✓ Medical compliance. People who are committed to following their doctor's advice and the band program do better.

The Dietitian's Assessment

Weight loss is the clear objective, but it is equally important that each patient maintain adequate nutrition as they lose. Most of us give little thought to the actual nutritional value of the foods we eat, and even if we do think about nutrition, we are often misinformed as to what our requirements are and which foods are best. Perhaps the most important assessment prior to surgery is the one you will have with a licensed and registered dietitian. It will involve an extensive dietary history, including not only what you eat but also when, where, and why. This information provides important insight as to which eating behaviors have been most responsible for the development of obesity in the first place.

The discussion with the dietitian may be somewhat uncomfortable for some patients. The probing questions asked may make you feel a sense of guilt, or even shame. While admitting certain eating habits to someone may be painful, it is a necessary part of the process of developing new habits. Say, for example, you make a habit of eating a whole box of cookies or a large bag of potato chips at one sitting. You know that habit has contributed to your weight problem, and you have vowed many times to stop. But now, when you are asked specific questions, you are embarrassed to admit it, so you simply withhold the information. After all, you know what to do, and you don't need somebody preaching to you about it, right? Well, don't you think if you really could change your behavior by yourself you would have done it already? The dietitian is trained to help you but will be unable to assist you change your behavior without full information.

During your evaluation by the dietitian, you may be tempted to demonstrate just how good you are at counting calories or how much you know about the basic food groups. A few patients have suggested that they know all about nutrition and don't really see the point of meeting with a dietitian. While your knowledge of nutrition may be considerable, each of us tends to be extraordinarily poor at evaluating our own behavior when it comes to food. So before you blow off this evaluation, recognize this as your opportunity to begin actually getting the help you need to change the food choices and eating habits that helped create and perpetuate your obesity. Just as with the psychological evaluation, you need to make every effort to answer the dietitian's questions as honestly as you can. To do any less is only cheating yourself.

After the dietitian has taken your dietary history, he or she will give you a thorough explanation of what and how you can expect to eat after the band is placed. This is an extremely important part of the dietitian's role. You can expect to eat more slowly, take smaller bites, chew your food thoroughly, and avoid drinking liquids during your meals. We have devoted an entire chapter to the subject, but suffice it to say that your success with the AGB program depends on your willingness to make a major commitment to modify your eating behavior.

Grace Ann's Story

I always thought my weight was about the bad habits I was taught as a child. I never could understand why my eating something would keep a baby from starving in another country. But my grandmother said it would. So I ate everything put in front of me. However, when I had my daughter, she totally blew my idea. I thought I could make her thin by never telling her to clean her plate. But it didn't work. My daughter as an adult is 300 pounds. There is no doubt in my mind that this weight problem is at least in part genetic.

My heart surgeon told me that I needed to lose weight. My top weight was 292 at 5-foot, 3/4-inch tall, and that was after my open heart surgery. At that weight, I was miserable. I couldn't move, my legs were so sore from swelling, and I felt like everything was too tight and cutting off my circulation. But really, it was my skin, stretched to the limit, that was cutting off my circulation. It was ugly. It was difficult.

Recently my husband and I joined Weight Watchers and paid our money. Then we had a death in the family and a bunch of other stuff going on. At the end of the Weight Watchers time we'd signed up for, we had each gained 6 pounds.

I ultimately decided I had to do something different. I've been banded for only three months now, and I've lost only 10 pounds. But already, I wouldn't go back. I thought I'd lose faster, but this is so much easier than dieting. With other weight-loss programs, I'd get so sick of what I was eating and I'd ask myself, "Am I supposed to do this all the time?" The biggest thing for me about the band is just knowing I can eat like this for the rest of my life. For example, I've had one hamburger in the last six weeks, something prohibited on other diets. I didn't eat all of it, but I probably could have. Now with food left over on my plate from a meal out, I can either give it away or save it for another meal, and that's okay. Before, if I went out to eat and brought food home, I just brought it home for show—I ate it as soon as I got home.

Another change is that I'm exercising and I have a personal trainer. I never felt like doing that before.

I live several hours from my surgeon, so I found a fill doctor only an hour away. My surgeon's office said they'd work with the fill doctor, but there was a misunderstanding about the type of band I had. I've gotten three fills but didn't feel as much restriction as I'd like. Turns out I had a bigger band than the fill doctor knew about. Also, my surgeon turned my post-op care over to another doctor who billed me extra for visiting me in the hospital. Since I'm a self-pay patient, I felt like these issues around my fills and the second doctor cost me additional money that wasn't necessary.

I do love the band. It is always there. I don't fall off the wagon and stay off like I did with diets. If I continue at this rate, I'll have all the weight I want off in a couple of years. But another problem I have encountered is there is not a band support group where I live, and, as I mentioned, my surgeon is several hours away by car. So I'm looking for other band people who can help me.

The Exercise Physiologist's Assessment

Increasing the level of physical activity is vital to success with any weight-loss program. This is particularly true with the AGB. However, it is obvious that getting regular exercise when you are significantly overweight can be a challenge, not only physically but also psychologically.

Virtually every patient we see has been on some type of exercise program in the past. Many have had personal trainers and have joined a local fitness center, often more than one. They have been told repeatedly that if they would just exercise regularly they will eventually lose weight. Personal trainers tend to be exercise fanatics, and many have a difficult time relating to the problems of someone who is morbidly obese. Not surprisingly they promote, and are usually excited to get you started on, the exercise routines that have worked for them. But, despite all the encouragement in the world, the absence of significant weight loss after hours of toiling away on some machine can often have a profoundly negative psychological impact. Many people just give up. It is simply too hard.

There is another group of fitness gurus that are involved in aggressive mass marketing of various products or exercise regimens that are "easy to do." "You too can have the body you've always wanted in as little as 10 minutes a day." Does it sound too good to be true? Obviously, they want you to buy their product. The professional models seem to move through the exercise effortlessly, and they don't even break a sweat. It's interesting that you never see advertisements for any exercise products showing a morbidly obese person actually using the device. In fact, in some cases the equipment may actually have a weight limit that prohibits its use if you weigh more than a certain amount.

As soon as the subject of exercise is brought up, many patients are quick to point out that they just can't do it. Obviously, morbid obesity often severely impairs an individual's physical capabilities. That is especially true with chronic back, hip, knee, ankle, or foot pain. This is why it is so important to work with someone who is experienced in recognizing these various restrictions, and who can develop specific physical activities that will increase metabolism and help burn off fat without aggravating underlying conditions. An exercise physiologist is trained to identify those ailments that restrict physical movement, and can develop an exercise program that you can actually do. Even patients with severe physical limitations that confine them to a wheelchair can be taught exercises they can readily do.

While weight in pounds is the most recognized measurement of obesity, it often does not reflect your true physical situation. Part of the preoperative assessment by an exercise physiologist is to obtain other specific measurements and perform an evaluation of your relative ability to participate in regular exercise. By obtaining a more comprehensive set of body measurements and assessing your exercise tolerance, the exercise physiologist will develop a more complete picture of how obesity is affecting your health. This initial data also provides an important baseline, and the same measurements will be repeated over the coming months and years to measure your success beyond just pounds lost. Many of my patients have gained significant encouragement from the inches they've lost, especially if they've hit a plateau regarding their weight. This initial assessment is part of your preparation for success and encouragement later.

Interacting with the exercise physiologist prior to surgery is also very important from a psychological standpoint. As has been repeatedly stated, some type of regular exercise is vital to your success, and virtually everyone will agree to exercise more provided they can have the AGB surgery. Unfortunately, these commitments are often rather vague and are quickly forgotten. What is required is a defined plan that outlines precisely what your exercise program is going to entail. Then you need to commit to it. This involves still another specific behavior modification, and is one of many lifestyle modifications, all of which involve also changing your thought process.

What about Obesity Surgery for Teens?

In the last few years the subject of bariatric surgery in morbidly obese children and adolescents has been discussed extensively in the media as well as within the medical and surgical community. The problem of childhood obesity is growing at an alarming rate, and all forecasts suggest that the situation is getting worse by the day. The anticipated health costs for dealing with obese kids as they become obese adults is staggering. Likewise, the psychological and social impact of childhood obesity has become a major issue among child psychologists. The obvious question is, Should we treat teenage obesity the same way we treat adult obesity, with surgery? Well, the jury is still out, but more and more pediatric surgeons are at least looking at this option.

When considering treating adolescent obesity with an operation, there are several questions that must be asked. These are the following: Are we sure the child is going to remain obese through and beyond puberty? Are we sure the child is mature enough to understand the ramifications of bariatric surgery and the restrictions it imposes? Is the child capable of dealing emotionally and socially with what may be a newfound "celebrity status" among their peers? And what procedure is appropriate for a person who is still developing physically?

Checklist: Questions to Ask before
Surgically Treating Adolescent Obesity

- ✓ Are we sure the child is going to remain obese through and beyond puberty?
- ✓ Are we sure the child is mature enough to understand the ramifications of bariatric surgery and the restrictions it imposes?
- ✓ Is the child capable of dealing emotionally and socially with what may be a newfound "celebrity status" among their peers?
- ✓ What procedure is appropriate for a person who is still developing physically?

There seems to be little doubt that if a person is obese as a child they are very likely to be obese as an adult. Many of my patients relate that they actually began gaining weight in their preteen years and have struggled with obesity their entire life. Certainly, a case can be made for intervening early in this process, before major medical problems, such as high blood pressure and diabetes, become well established. However, it is hard to know when and if these problems will actually develop, when surgical intervention is warranted, and when it isn't. After all, we aren't dealing with a long medical history, since by definition these are children we are talking about.

Another argument that is frequently made suggests that teens who are morbidly obese suffer from impaired social development, so obviously they should benefit from bariatric surgery as a psychosocial development tool. Unfortunately, most children under the age of 18 have limited insight into their psychosocial situation and are generally most comfortable maintaining the status quo. They are often quite uncomfortable drawing undue attention to themselves, especially if it involves their appearance. Assessing the child's motivations and likely response to a major change in body image is perhaps the most critical part of any adolescent bariatric program. One program I'm familiar with requires one full year of psychological assessment and counseling before any child is considered a candidate for surgery. It is also extremely important to identify the motivations and the role of the parents in this process. The decision to explore weight management through surgery must be shared by both child and parents if there is any hope for success.

We all know how important "image" is, especially to a child around the age of puberty. Assuming that a high school student who is recognized by their peers as the "big man" or "big girl" on campus suddenly begins to lose a large amount of weight, they will undoubtedly become the subject of considerable interest, some positive and some negative. This unusual level of attention can potentially cause a number of problems. They may achieve sudden "star" status, or sudden "freak" status. Either way can lead to a variety of behavioral changes, including juvenile delinquency, poor performance in school, and even drug use. Children who undergo bariatric surgery must be followed very closely by an experienced child psychologist or psychiatrist to help identify such behaviors before they become a serious problem. These kids should also be compelled to be involved in a support group of their peers as well as a supervised exercise program.

If a well-adjusted, emotionally stable, morbidly obese child and their parents make the decision to have weight-loss surgery, it only makes sense to employ the lowest risk procedure possible, and preferably one that is reversible. It is certainly possible that within the next few decades one or more medical treatments will come along in the form of a new diet pill or a genetic re-engineering process that may make bariatric surgery obsolete. Should that occur, it might be advantageous to reverse whatever weight-loss procedure a young man or woman may have had performed when they were an adolescent.

The entire subject of bariatric surgery in children remains very controversial, but it is one that will continue to spark considerable debate in the years to come. At this time, if any parent is considering bariatric surgery for their child, they should first seek the advice of their pediatrician. It is also important to recognize that there are only a handful of centers capable of providing all the special testing and care required to be successful. Remember, children have special needs. They are not just small adults.

Conclusion

Assuming you are a candidate for the AGB, your overall success will depend on many factors, beyond the operation itself. The complexity of obesity as a disease requires more than just an operation. In the next chapter, we'll look into why you need a comprehensive approach to treat your obesity and what you should be looking for in the way of a program.

7

What Does a Comprehensive AGB Program Look Like?

*I don't want any yes-men around me. I want everybody
to tell me the truth even if it costs them their jobs.*
—Samuel Goldwyn, movie producer

Someone asked me the other day about getting a band. The first thing I said was, "You realize it isn't really about surgery, right?" The look I got back was one of total surprise. After all, they had read about "the surgery" on the Internet, they knew someone who had actually had "the surgery," and they saw an ad in the newspaper about how much weight some guy had lost after "the surgery." The procedure certainly sounds safe enough. After years of struggling with weight, it seems like a miracle cure. So, of course, "I want one, too." Armed with this certainty, some people are even willing to fly off to a foreign country to have someone they have never even met before, and will probably never see again, put a band around their stomach. Simple–right? Well . . . no!

People are drawn to having bariatric surgery for a variety of reasons but nearly always with a sense of finality. In many respects it represents a last resort approach to losing weight. I've heard many patients say, "I've tried everything else, so this just has to work." There is clearly a sense of desperation, which in many cases is accompanied by a transfer of responsibility for success, or failure, directly to the surgery. But surgery alone, no matter what kind of operation, cannot solve the problem by itself. Let me give you an example.

A woman approached me after a seminar a few years back, inquiring about whether she would be a candidate for the band procedure. She weighed about

350 pounds, so I thought she would surely meet our criteria. However, she went on to tell me that 25 years earlier she'd had a gastric bypass operation and had lost 175 pounds. Over the next several years she gained all her weight back again. What that meant to me is that through consistent overeating she had stretched out the stomach pouch that had been created by the bypass, and was able to overeat the way she had before her surgery. She went on to say that 10 years ago she had another operation to revise her stomach pouch, meaning that the surgeon had essentially redone the gastric bypass. Again she lost 175 pounds, only to regain it all yet again over the next few years. Now she was looking to the AGB. I'd like to say that was the only time I'd heard such a story, but it's not. For me, stories like this woman's are extreme examples of how surgery alone doesn't solve the problem.

Do I Really Need a Weight Management Program?

Getting a band should be viewed as merely the first step toward making major and permanent changes in your lifestyle. Changing the way you eat, what you eat, the role that food plays in your life, how and when you exercise, even how you view yourself are all part of the road to success. The fact is that all of these things and more must change. One of my favorite quotes is from Albert Einstein: "Insanity is doing the same thing over and over and expecting different results."

You have to change the way you behave, not just go get an operation. The question is, Can you make those changes alone? It has been my experience that very few people are capable of the degree of self-analysis, self-direction, and self-motivation required to make lifestyle changes without some help.

As we discussed in a previous chapter, the band is a tool, but like any tool it requires proper instruction in its use. No virtuoso pianist just sat down one day and began playing a Chopin concerto. To get the most out of any tool requires not only instruction and practice but also oversight and continued guidance. Call it coaching, if you will. The band is a tremendous device, capable of producing wonderful results when used appropriately by a well-motivated patient, but to obtain consistent and long-lasting success requires a team approach, and even then the battle is not easily won. Conquering a lifetime of obesity is a formidable task that requires both your personal commitment and a team of professionals dedicated to helping you achieve your goal. It is critical that you and your team have a coordinated plan that you understand and agree to follow. This is what I mean by A PROGRAM. The surgeon, dietitian, an exercise physiologist, and psychologists each play their separate but equally important parts within a comprehensive weight-loss program.

The Surgeon

In the last chapter, we discussed appropriate criteria for patients seeking the adjustable gastric band. Assuming that those criteria are met, the next step is finding a surgeon and a comprehensive program. Whether you find the program first and work with a surgeon they recommend, or find a surgeon who has developed a program—it doesn't really matter. What does matter is that you have both, a reputable surgeon and a comprehensive program.

Finding someone capable and willing to do band surgery was a problem in the early days of the AGB in the United States. Today there are many more surgeons performing these operations, and advertisements for the procedure can be found almost everywhere. So how do you know who to go to? Is it enough to go to a doctor just because your friend went there? Should you assume they did their homework and found the best surgeon and the best program? The answer to these questions should be obvious. For something as important as this, you should do your own research, even to the point of interviewing several surgeons before you decide.

The first question you should ask the surgeon or the office staff is, Are you part of a comprehensive program? If you call a surgeon's office and ask about their program, and they act as if they don't know what you are talking about, then the answer is clearly no. If their answer is "Yes, we have a support group that meets once a month," you should probe further. What you are looking for is a clearly defined program that offers nutritional, exercise, and psychological support and guidance from true professionals. Don't hesitate to ask plenty of questions. Find out how adjustments are done and who performs them, what kind of nutritional counseling they offer, what psychological support is available, whether they provide exercise guidance, and what the follow-up process is. Even if the surgeon doesn't have a formal program, he or she should still have made some arrangement for patients to receive all of these necessary services.

Checklist: Questions to Ask before Choosing a Surgeon and a Program

✓ Is the surgeon part of a comprehensive program? (If they don't know what that means, you have your answer.)
✓ Does the surgeon have a patient support group?
✓ How are adjustments done, and who does them?
✓ What kind of nutritional counseling is available?
✓ What psychological support is available?

✓ Does the surgeon provide exercise guidance, and what is the follow-up process?

✓ Are these services provided by trained professionals? (You're looking for licensed dietitians, exercise physiologists, and psychologists.)

✓ Ask about your surgeon's experience with laparoscopic techniques. Is the surgeon experienced with laparoscopic suturing? Is the surgeon certified through the American Society of General Surgeons PALSS program?

✓ What about patients who haven't done well or who are failing to lose weight? What percentage of patients are struggling, and what's been done to help them succeed?

✓ What kind of complications have there been? (You're looking for infections, slippage, and band erosion as the most common complications.)

✓ Ask the surgeon to explain the common complications, what he or she does to help prevent them, and how they are handled when they occur.

✓ Ask yourself, How comfortable do I feel?

Provided the surgeon has or is affiliated with an adequate program, your next questions should be about training, experience, and results. In 1988 the world of surgery changed forever. That was the year that laparoscopic surgery in the United States really got started. Since then many different operations have been performed using this revolutionary technique; however, it is important to recognize that not all surgeons have embraced this technique for doing abdominal surgery. Many have little experience beyond the removal of the gallbladder or the appendix. It is only in the last few years that laparoscopic surgery has been taught to any extent in surgical training programs, and many of those who are "teaching" these techniques have only limited experience themselves.

There is a new laparoscopic skills certification process offered by the American Society of General Surgeons called PALSS, which stands for Proficiency Assessment of Laparoscopic Surgical Skills. This certification is a peer review evaluation of laparoscopic skills, and it may offer patients some level of assurance that their surgeon has demonstrated his or her technical ability to a panel of experts. The program is still in its early development and as such is not yet considered a benchmark in the surgical community. Only a few surgeons have actually participated in the PALSS program so far, but it is a start.

The American Society of Bariatric Surgeons has also put together a process for designating facilities as "Centers of Excellence" in bariatric surgery. Typically these are hospitals or surgical centers that do a large number of bariatric procedures. Such a designation is more a reflection of the number of procedures done in that facility than it is the individual experience of a specific surgeon. While having an experienced staff with all the necessary equipment and services available at the facility is an important aspect of your care, the surgeon is the most important part of the equation. Just because a facility or even the individual surgeon does a huge volume of business is no assurance of the quality of the service you are likely to receive.

The laparoscopic placement of an adjustable gastric band is generally considered to be a fairly advanced procedure that requires significant laparoscopic skills—in particular, the ability to place sutures. You should not hesitate to ask the surgeon about their training and experience with laparoscopic suturing. Even if he or she hasn't performed thousands of banding procedures, the surgeon may possess the necessary skills, provided they have experience with other advanced laparoscopic operations. You may want to ask the surgeon about his or her experience with hiatal hernia repairs, antireflux operations, colon resections, and other procedures that they perform using the laparoscopic technique. Any reputable surgeon will be happy to share their experience with you. If the answer you get indicates that sutures are either unnecessary or unimportant, that should tell you everything you need to know.

During your interview, you should also ask the surgeon about results. Don't accept an answer that simply quotes the latest medical literature. You need to know what kind of results your surgeon is getting. Every surgeon will have some patients who are doing extremely well, and naturally those are the ones that you are likely to hear about first. Make sure to inquire about those whose results have been less than satisfactory. If the surgeon has been doing the AGB procedure for any length of time, he or she will have some failures. Find out why the surgeon thinks those particular patients failed to achieve their objective and what has been done to help improve their results.

You should also ask about complications, such as infections, band slippage, and erosions. The surgeon will likely provide you with information about potential risks even before you ask, but don't hesitate to inquire further if you are not satisfied with the information you get. This subject is covered more thoroughly later in the chapter on complications, but make sure you understand them directly from your surgeon.

Personally, I think that one of the most important criteria when deciding on a surgeon is how comfortable you feel. All the credentials in the world or affiliations with the most prestigious medical centers are no substitute for the feeling of confidence you get following a face-to-face meeting. Some bariatric practices are so busy and so automated that the surgeon doesn't actually see the patient until just before the operation. This time-saving process may be fine for the surgeon, but it is rather impersonal. You should insist on a personal meeting before you commit to anything, and you should specifically discuss the procedure, and all the other issues mentioned earlier, directly with the surgeon. If you are told that is not possible, or if the meeting is only a brief "Hi, how are you?" then you should probably go elsewhere.

Nutritional Support

The whole idea of having a band around your stomach is to alter the amount of food you can eat. But with that kind of restriction, there is a need to ensure that the food you eat has adequate nutritional value. Getting enough protein, vitamins, and minerals can be a real challenge. Somewhat surprisingly, it can also be difficult to drink enough water. Failure to take in the right things in the right amounts can lead to a variety of problems, so the assistance of a professional dietitian throughout the process is essential.

Any bariatric program will likely have some form of nutritional counseling after the procedure, but it is important that this individual, or group of individuals, also be part of the initial screening process before surgery. Prospective patients need to hear ahead of time precisely what they can expect to eat and what changes they will need to make in the way they eat.

For the band patient it isn't just a matter of eating the "right stuff." Having a band requires you to eat differently, and many patients find changing their eating habits to be the most difficult part of the program. If you are unwilling or unable to change the way you eat, your results will be disappointing to say the least. There can be no substitute for proper instruction by someone who understands the way the band works, followed by positive feedback when these changes are actually achieved.

This difficult task of instructing, challenging, and encouraging the patient is done largely by the dietitian. The need for professional guidance is especially critical for patients with Type 2 diabetes, because their blood sugars and subsequent medication requirements can, and frequently do, change even more rapidly than their weight.

Finally, the dietitian also needs to be involved in the process of deciding when and to what degree adjustments are made to the tightness of the band. Having the dietitian's input is very important. A well-trained professional can usually see through the protests of the patient, and help the patient recognize that it may not be the tightness of the band that is creating problems as much as it is their own reluctance to change the way they eat. For the band patient, the dietitian must be part psychologist, part nutritionist, part drill sergeant, part den mother, and part coach. But most of all the dietitian must stay involved, especially during the first year, when those new eating habits are being created.

Sue's Story

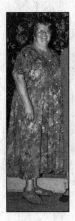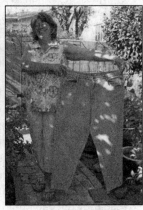

(Left) Sue, pre-op, 312 pounds.

(Right) Sue, four years post-op, 185 pounds, holding jeans that used to fit tightly.

I was 53 years old, 312 pounds at 5 feet, 8 inches, and my quality of life was lousy. In fact, I was pretty sure I wasn't going to live much longer. What made it worse was I taught preschool and felt the principal was prejudiced against overweight people. Plus I had sleep apnea and was on a C-pap machine, and I had knee and hip pain.

I tried the usual diets, including Jenny Craig® and Weight Watchers®. When those didn't work I did a ton of research on surgery. My insurance would cover the bypass but not the band. But the mortality rates for the gastric bypass really scared me. I felt I'd be crippled or die before I had the time to save the money to have the surgery in the States, and back then there was a much bigger difference. So I had the surgery in Mexico.

I had a huge case of buyer's regret afterward. My experience in Mexico was fine, and I was supposed to go to a hotel after a few hours. But I had some residual esophageal swelling, so they kept me overnight. After they released me I went home, but the swelling didn't go down enough and I was getting really dehydrated. After a couple of days, I even stopped producing saliva. It was hot. I live in California. I was sweating. I had to carry a cup around to spit into because my own spit wouldn't stay down and I couldn't sleep. I called the doctor in Mexico and he suggested I come back, but I didn't want to. I didn't think I could make it back to Mexico. I wasn't even peeing anymore at that point.

So the Mexico doctor found a U.S. doctor near me and got me admitted to their ER. I spent four days in the hospital on IVs. They checked the band to see if it had slipped, but I was fine. I think that would have happened no matter where I got the band. I didn't have a fill for almost a year. I didn't need one. And I lost a lot of weight. Now I'm at 185.

When I did get a fill, I found a U.S. doctor and got a very small one to start with. I'm not real thrilled with driving around on the other side of the border. My husband is a police officer, and he's really cautious. It's just too much of a pain to go back.

I don't feel hungry anymore. I have to remind myself to eat. At midday I have to eat some lunch so I don't eat too much at dinner. I remember having my stomach growl and the feeling I would eat anything that doesn't move.

There are some things I'll never eat again, such as pizza crust or toast. But if I start feeling deprived I go to my closet and say, Is the toast worth being where I was? No way. I remember I used to lie down on the bed and suck my stomach in to zip and button the pants I'm holding in the "after" photo.

There are other things. I flew to see my daughter on the East Coast right after 9–11, and I had no room. I could barely wedge myself into the airline seat. It was torture. Two years later I got on the plane to see her again, and I put the tray table down. I could cross my legs. I thought, This is heaven. I go to amusement parks now and I ride the rides. I used to have to stand and watch. Some rides I don't do because they're scary, but I can if I want to. Last summer I went to Colorado and climbed up Pikes Peak. I also went to New Mexico and climbed up some ruins. I can do more now than I could when I was in my late forties.

I look in the mirror and think I need plastic surgery. But I'm not doing that. My arms are real hangy, but so what? I'd like to have the roll around my stomach gone, but I don't know that I will. No one sees it. I don't run around in shorts or bathing suits. And now that I'm retired, I don't think it matters.

My only regret now is that I didn't do this years ago. I lost so much of my life. I wish it had been more widely available in the United States. And I like it that the band is reversible. I could go back because my anatomy hasn't changed, although I wouldn't want to now.

An Exercise Program

Joining a health club or getting a personal trainer may be precisely what some people need to develop an exercise program and remain committed to it. But if that's all it took to be successful in losing weight, you would not be reading this book. To some extent the failure of exercise programs alone in dealing with obesity may be related to the fact that many personal trainers have little training and experience with obesity and the physical limitations that go along with it. Morbidly obese individuals are frequently unable to do the kind of exercises that the typical personal trainer expects. Another aspect that can lead to failure is the psychological impact of "going to the gym." It often seems that everyone else who is there is trying to get "buff," while you are just trying to survive. "Is it my imagination, or is everybody really here just to watch me struggle?" Not surprisingly, some obese people decide they are just not going back because of the humiliation factor.

Despite the pain, and the embarrassment, getting some form of exercise is critical to your success. Exercise increases your metabolism and burns off fat stores that would otherwise remain despite dieting. A comprehensive program needs to have someone who is experienced in both the physiology of exercise and the special needs of obese patients. It is important to develop an exercise routine that is not only effective at increasing your metabolic rate but also safe, given the physical limitations that obesity may impose. This role is very different from that of a personal trainer, and is one that is more appropriately filled by an experienced exercise physiologist or physical therapist. It also doesn't require daily or even weekly instruction. This type of exercise specialist can provide patients with directions for developing a gradually evolving exercise regimen using only periodic encounters.

Part of the preoperative evaluation process should be an interview with the exercise physiologist or physical therapist that will help establish their role as part of the program. This includes a formal assessment of the patient's physical condition and limitations, as well as an evaluation of the patient's preoperative exercise tolerance. Recommendations are made as to what kinds of exercise are appropriate and safe.

A complete set of body measurements, such as chest, waist, hips, arms, legs, and neck, should also be performed as part of the general physical assessment. Despite the fact that some patients find these measurements embarrassing, they actually provide one of the most important motivations and feedback mechanisms in the whole program. Once every three months these same measurements are repeated, and patients can see just how many inches they have lost around their waist, hips, thighs, and every other area measured. It is a universal source of delight and inspiration, often even more so than the number of pounds lost. I've seen many patients proudly carrying their measurements around like a "straight A report card." They are eager to show everyone just how successful they are. Armed with their documented success, they become even more excited about the prospect of expanding their exercise routine so that by the next time they are measured the results will be even greater.

Changing How You Think

It seems as though individual success in our society is often measured by our ability to be self-sufficient, self-motivated, and able to "pull ourselves up by the boot straps." We place great emphasis on "the will to win" and the power of that will. We are made to believe that the difference between failure and success is a strong mind, capable of controlling behavior in every situation. Conversely, we conclude that anyone who would allow their weight to get out of control is weak-minded and undisciplined or just plain lazy. Clearly these assumptions and conclusions are wrong.

If you ask anyone who has been involved in bariatric surgery for any length of time, they will tell you that the psychological aspects of obesity are perhaps the most important and certainly the most challenging. A big part of the challenge comes from the social and psychological stigma that seems to go along with obesity. The mere suggestion that a psychological assessment needs to be done before undergoing bariatric surgery can solicit a defensive response, such as "I'm not crazy!" or, "I certainly don't think I need a shrink!" Along that same line, I've even seen professionals who anticipate a negative reaction from the patient and start by making excuses for the request for a psychological evaluation even before the patient has had an opportunity to raise any objections.

The real reason for our reluctance to submit to an analysis of our thoughts and our behaviors is often fear. There is nothing more personal or more private than our thoughts, especially as they relate to how we perceive ourselves. To have someone probing into our thoughts and perceptions naturally makes us feel uncomfortable, vulnerable, and exposed. But to be successful at changing a lifetime of self-destructive behavior, we must first change the way we think. We have to identify self-defeating, negative thoughts before we can replace them with the positive thoughts that will lead to changes in our behavior. This requires professional help.

A comprehensive weight management program should include an initial assessment by a clinical psychologist or psychiatrist trained in the science of human behavior. This evaluation may be in the form of a standardized test or a personal interview, or preferably both. The objective of this assessment is to determine whether the patient is capable of participating in the program and the patient's receptiveness to change. Occasionally this evaluation will uncover specific personality traits that make the patient destined to struggle with changing behavior, and it is far better to find this out before any surgical procedure is done. In addition, as covered in Chapter 6, insurance programs often require patients to receive a psychological evaluation before weight-loss surgery.

But the psychological components of a comprehensive program go far beyond the initial evaluation. They encompass a whole group of behavior modification tools, not all of which are provided by the psychologist. The elements of a psychological support system range from something as simple as a regular newsletter that provides specific direction and positive testimonials, to a series of formal behavior modification sessions conducted by a clinical psychologist. Actually, every member of the team plays a critical role in supporting patients during their struggle to regain control over their lives. Routine office visits with the dietitian, the surgeon, and even the exercise physiologist should include positive reinforcement of the patient's evolving behaviors. As Steven Greer, Ph.D., mentioned in Chapter 6, under *What We Look for in Psychological Testing of AGB Patients*, the psychological evaluation can help the team by supplying them with information critical to helping the patient succeed.

Five Steps to Changing Your Thinking
G. Dick Miller, Psychologist

There are five steps to changing your thinking. The first step is to become an observer of yourself. One good way to do this is simply to write down what is in your head for a week or so. Don't judge it. Just record your inner dialogue. Personal honesty is the key—an honest look at what your beliefs are now. What is really happening in your own head? There's no need to beat yourself up. Just take a look.

The second step is to look to see if your thinking makes sense or if it's nonsense. The trick is to identify the thinking that isn't working. Everyone at one time or another has struggled with this. But it makes sense to check your beliefs. There are five simple rules you can compare your thinking with to see if you're beliefs are rational. They are: Is it literally true? Is it good for my physical health? Is the way I'm thinking now consistent with my short- and long-term goals? Does it prevent significant conflict with others? Does it help me feel the way I want to feel? "The Tests for Rational Beliefs" in Chapter 8 cover these five questions in more detail.

The third step is to come up with a new way of thinking that is rational. This is where you challenge your current mindset. For example, if you've been telling yourself that two cookies won't make a difference in your diet, then it's time to challenge that idea. Will two cookies make a difference? A "no" answer is not rational. Of course they do. They make a difference in your intake for the day, they can lead to permission to have more (after all, I already blew it), they affect your blood sugar, which can lead to ups and downs emotionally and physically, and they can lead to other problems as well; so two cookies do make a difference.

The fourth step is to practice. Start telling yourself what is rational. Use the new rational statement you've come up with to replace the old. So when the thought comes that two cookies don't make a difference, replace it with the thought that two cookies do make a difference. You can also add that you'd rather wake up tomorrow morning feeling good about yourself because you did what is in your own best interest.

The fifth step is learning to tolerate being uncomfortable. Whenever you do something new a pattern gets generated in your brain called "cognitive dissonance." What that means is that your brain is going to generate convictions like these: "This is weird," "It doesn't feel right," "I feel awkward,"

"I wonder if someone else thinks I'm stupid," and so on. In fact, cognitive dissonance occurs anytime you learn something new, from a golf swing to cooking a new recipe. I'd go as far as to say that if you don't feel uncomfortable, you're not doing something new at all, which means you're not making the necessary changes. The challenge is learning to tolerate discomfort—to give yourself time as you adjust to the change you're introducing in your life. Knowing you're going to experience this can be encouraging. You may actually begin to look forward to being uncomfortable because it's a sign you're making progress.

Checklist: Five Steps to Change

1. Observe your thinking—practice personal honesty.
2. Check your thinking against the five rules for rational thinking.
3. Challenge your beliefs—come up with a new way of thinking that is rational.
4. Practice the new thinking.
5. Tolerate being uncomfortable.

These five steps to change are your steps to success. And they can become a habit, one you can use to ensure your weight-loss using the band.

Summary of a Comprehensive Program

While losing a large amount of weight using only your own willpower can be done, it is pretty rare. Unfortunately, for the majority of people who struggle with obesity the problem and the solution are anything but simple. So being successful in losing weight, and in keeping it off, requires more than just a diet, or an exercise plan, or surgery, or even creating a positive mental image. It actually requires all of those components working together in a coordinated program, and more. The "more" is the dedication and hard work of the patient. No matter what anyone tells you, it isn't easy, even with a team of experts helping you. But the rewards can be generous. When asked about the program a year or two after surgery, many patients relate, "It's the best thing I have ever done for myself."

Once you have found a comprehensive program, the next step is often the hardest. It takes a great deal of courage to call for a doctor's appointment when the problem you are calling about is obesity. But, as is frequently said, "Every great journey begins with the first step." Making that step is up to you.

Medical Management of the AGB

8

What to Expect before Surgery

Life shrinks or expands in proportion to one's courage.
—Anais Nin, *The Diary of Anais Nin*

Patients always point to the day of their surgery with great expectation. It is, in fact, a major event, one that marks a life transition. But, before going to the operating room, there are a few details that should be addressed to help ensure your safety. In this chapter those details are examined, along with why they are important. Having a clear idea of what to expect can allay some fears and create an atmosphere of appropriate anticipation.

Pre-op Testing

Many patients have already had a thorough medical evaluation by their primary physician prior to being referred for weight-loss surgery. This is particularly true for patients with known medical problems such as diabetes, hypertension, and heart disease. But, for patients who have not seen their personal physician recently, some routine lab tests to determine their current health status may be necessary. Likewise, if questions or concerns arise about specific medical issues during the assessment process, specific tests may be required before proceeding with AGB surgery. In some instances, the results of these tests can actually determine whether the AGB is even a reasonable weight-loss option.

Since the operation requires general anesthesia, meaning you will be completely asleep and under the care of the anesthesiologist, the status of your cardiac and pulmonary functions is obviously important. For most patients this is relatively easy to determine through a medical history and examination. However, for those with a history of significant medical problems, it may be necessary to perform a more extensive evaluation of specific organs.

If there is a history of chronic respiratory problems, an evaluation of pulmonary function may be recommended. Patients with poor lung function, especially those who require oxygen even at rest, have a higher than usual risk during anesthesia. Armed with this information the anesthesiologist may request that a pulmonologist, or lung specialist, be called in prior to surgery to optimize the patient's breathing.

In the same way, patients with a history of heart problems may require a cardiology assessment to determine the relative risk of a cardiac complication during or after surgery. This may include an electrocardiogram, or in some cases a cardiac stress test, to see how the heart is likely to respond to the pressures of surgery.

Patients with diabetes should have their blood sugar under reasonable control before surgery, especially immediately prior to the procedure and immediately afterward. Blood glucose levels can change significantly as a result of many factors, including the preoperative diet, the absence of any food on the day of the procedure, intravenous fluids and medications, as well as the stress of surgery. Testing the blood glucose frequently during these times is relatively easy to do and provides important information for maintaining a safe operative course.

For patients with a history of liver or kidney disease, a comprehensive set of blood tests will provide a better picture of the functional status of those vital organs. If there is significant compromise of either organ system, it may not be advisable to proceed with surgery without consulting with an expert. For problems with kidney function that specialist would be a nephrologist, and for abnormal liver function the expert would be a gastroenterologist or hepatologist. Depending on the extent of the problem, as well as whether it is recent in onset or more chronic in nature, surgery to place the AGB may or may not be a reasonable choice.

One of the more common comorbidities that accompany obesity is sleep apnea. In some cases this may be the major reason why the patient is seeking weight-loss surgery. Many patients complain of severe snoring, problems sleeping, or chronic fatigue. These issues are often related to sleep apnea, but most patients with these symptoms have not undergone a formal sleep study. Those who have are usually on some form of airway support at night such as CPAP or BiPAP. Some have even undergone one or more surgical procedures to improve their airways.

While a sleep study can demonstrate the presence of sleep apnea, the question is whether confirming the diagnosis in this manner is going to change the procedure. The definitive treatment for sleep apnea is weight loss, which is obviously the objective of the AGB surgery. Sleep studies are often costly, and whether the outcome of the test is positive or negative isn't likely to change the planned procedure. The main reason for getting a sleep study prior to surgery is often to document the condition in an effort to satisfy insurance criteria for the surgery. If documenting sleep apnea is necessary, whatever the reason, there is no better test than an overnight sleep study. The test is best performed in a sleep laboratory equipped with extensive monitoring equipment. It can also be done in your own home, but the ability to monitor is generally more limited.

Although each of these preoperative tests can help offer you peace of mind, they are by no means a guarantee against serious complications. Even someone with no history of any previous medical problems could still have complications during surgery. The question is invariably raised as to whether every patient should undergo an extensive battery of tests prior to having any type of surgery. However, currently there is no evidence to suggest that such an approach would significantly change the outcome for most patients. The most important factors in reducing the risks of surgery are an experienced surgeon and anesthesiologist, along with an operating team that is familiar with the procedure and attentive to the details of your care.

The Pre-op Diet

Some doctors are willing to proceed directly to surgery once a patient is determined to be an appropriate candidate for the AGB. While it is generally possible to perform the procedure safely, this approach risks encountering situations that can make the operation far more difficult than it needs to be. Patients who are morbidly obese almost always have significant stores of a fatty material called glycogen in their liver. The livers of obese patients are often quite large and heavy, making it difficult to expose and perform the necessary dissection around the upper part of the stomach. The pre-op diet is designed to shrink the liver so that it's smaller and lighter, to make band surgery safer.

Preoperative Liver-Shrinking Diet

Provided by the MASTER CENTER® for Minimally Invasive Surgery— Texas, LLP

Three Week Nutrition Plan*
Goal: To decrease the size of the liver prior to AGB surgery.

Breakfast: High-protein drink supplement—2 scoops
(300 calories and 48 grams of protein)
See "Recipes for Protein Shakes" on pages 144–145

Lunch: High-protein drink supplement—2 scoops
(300 calories and 48 grams of protein)
See "Recipes for Protein Shakes" on pages 144–145

Dinner: Broiled, baked, or grilled chicken, fish, or turkey (4 oz. cooked—28 grams of protein)
  Low-calorie vegetables (2 cups), such as green beans, carrots, broccoli, celery, spinach, beets, tomatoes, cauliflower, brussels sprouts, turnip greens, asparagus, zucchini squash, yellow squash, cabbage, cucumbers, radishes, eggplant, or okra (boiled).
  Salad: Lettuce and tomato; fat-free salad dressing
  Fresh fruit—1 cup
  (400 calories)

Snack: (200 calories)
  See Protein snack list on page 146

---

*See your dietitian or doctor to adjust your protein intake if you experience fluid retention coupled with a rise in blood pressure, fatigue, nausea, and/or loss of appetite, or if an increase in calories is needed.

The size of the fatty liver can be significantly decreased by placing the patient on a pre-op diet designed to use up the glycogen stored in the liver, effectively shrinking it and making it easier to move out of the way during surgery. In my practice, our dietitian places each patient on a low-fat, low-carbohydrate diet for three weeks before surgery. The diet consists of a protein shake for two meals each day. The third meal consists of broiled or grilled fish, chicken, or turkey accompanied by vegetables without added fat such as butter or margarine.

Virtually everyone can stay on this diet for three weeks as long as they understand what we are trying to accomplish. Typically patients lose 8 to 10 pounds during this time, which provides them with a great positive head start to their program.

The Tests for Rational Beliefs

G. Dick Miller, Psychologist

As I've already mentioned, challenging your current beliefs is the way to change your thinking. After you have written down what you're thinking about food and what you are eating, you can use these five tests to see if what you are telling yourself is rational. There is nothing new about these principles. If you examine your thinking with these rules, and replace erroneous beliefs with ones that line up with these principles, you'll find yourself on the way to making the changes you want to see in your weight.

The first test is a simple one: Is it literally true? In other words, Could I defend this statement to someone impartial? I am often called as an expert witness in court, and my daughter is an attorney. At times I tell her I am concerned about a certain case, that I'm not sure I am as prepared as I should be. She says, "Just get up there, tell them the facts, and shut up." That is a rule to use talking to myself, not just to a jury.

The second test: Is it good for my physical health? Many people will consistently rationalize thinking and the resulting actions that are inconsistent with their physical health. Often we are talking about the chemicals we put in our body. Our grandparents didn't have to make this decision. They grew what they ate, the quantity was limited, and there weren't preservatives, junk food, or stores on wheels. I hear statements like "So everybody drinks," or "What is one cookie going to matter?"

What we find out when we examine those thoughts is that everyone doesn't have bad habits when it comes to food. Now I'll grant you that more of us have bad habits because of the culture we live in. But our choices do catch up with us. Really, everyone doesn't do it, and do you want to be one of those who does?

The third test: Is the way I am thinking right now consistent with my short- and long-term goals? I think it becomes clear when I have people write their homework assignments dialoging their inner conversation. It's clear that we sell ourselves out for our short-term goals at the expense of our long-term goals. If you ask someone if they want good health when they're older, they will say yes. But with the help from Madison Avenue and our history of irrational thinking, we're not making choices that work for both our short-term and long-term goals. I often find myself thinking, "I'm a good guy. I deserve that cake or drink I want." But if I look at my long-term goals, I see that it's more important to lose weight, to live longer, to be here for my grandchildren. It is a smart decision to take both sets of goals into account, because if I act exclusively in terms of my short-term goals, I can set myself up to suffer long term.

The fourth test is: Does it prevent significant conflict with others? This doesn't apply as much with food, because abusing food, unlike alcohol or drugs, does not usually put me in conflict with others. But think about how able you'll be to participate with your friends and grandkids if you continue to gain weight. And what about conflict with yourself? Each person knows what they've done. Even if the food disappears and no one saw you eat it, you know. How do you feel about that?

The fifth and final test is this: Does it help me feel the way I want to feel? I can ask myself, "Will what I'm putting in my mouth make me feel better?" It might, short term, if it's sugar or alcohol. But what about the resulting crash later? Is this really the best choice for feeling the way you want to feel?

Checklist: The Five Tests for Rational Beliefs

Write down your thoughts, then check them against this list.

1. Is it literally true?
2. Is it good for my physical health?
3. Is the way I'm thinking now consistent with my short- and long-term goals?
4. Does it prevent significant conflict with others?
5. Does it help me feel the way I want to feel?

These five tests for rational thinking are the basis of acting responsibly. Realistically, you may be able to act contrary to your belief systems for a while, but if you don't change the way you think, sooner or later your behavior is going to line up with your thinking. As you can probably see, personal honesty is the key here. If you look at your thinking, evaluate it, challenge it with these guidelines, practice the new way of thinking, and tolerate feeling uncomfortable during the transition period, you can and will succeed. But if you decide you're being forced to do something you don't want to do, if you make changing your thinking into a "have to" task instead of a "want to," then your chances at success diminish. We'll look at the "have to" mentality next.

Just before Surgery

Before surgery I have patients come into the office for a last preoperative visit. That is when we see just how well they have done on the preoperative diet. We go over the sequence of events that are going to happen on the day of surgery, and make sure that any last-minute questions are answered. I give each patient prescriptions and encourage them to get them filled prior to the day of their surgery. That way they won't be running around trying to find a pharmacy on their way home from the hospital. The prescriptions include a medication for pain (usually a liquid rather than a pill), as well as antinausea medication.

Our patients are also advised to prepare for their homecoming by stocking up on the foods they are going to need after surgery. The dietitian gives each patient a postoperative diet to follow for the first few weeks after the band is placed, but they really need to stock up only on the food they will need for the first few days. This includes things like sugar-free liquids, Jell-O, low-calorie puddings, and a liquid protein supplement.

Hospitals can be somewhat intimidating places, so to be better prepared, I recommend a preoperative visit to the hospital a few days before the procedure. The nursing staff will show you around and provide specific instructions as to where you should go and what time you should arrive on the day of your surgery. Any preoperative blood tests may also be drawn at that time. You'll also be told not to eat or drink anything past a certain hour (usually midnight) before your operation. This helps ensure that your stomach is empty at the time of surgery.

A meeting with the anesthesiologist is a very important part of your preoperative preparation. He or she will need to be familiar with your medical history prior to putting you to sleep. They will be particularly interested in knowing if you've ever had any problems with anesthesia before, or if you have family members who have had problems with anesthesia. Be sure and share that information.

Ideally this should be a face-to-face discussion, but the fact is that anesthesiologists don't generally have regular office hours. Instead, they try to see patients at the hospital between cases. Unfortunately, they are frequently busy giving anesthesia to other patients during the time when preoperative patients are visiting the hospital. So if you don't have the opportunity to meet the anesthesiologist, you can make arrangements to have a personal contact by phone a day or two before your surgery. You will also get a chance to meet and visit with your anesthesiologist just prior to the operation.

As part of the routine preoperative procedure, you'll be asked to sign several documents. These may include a general Consent to Treat form that simply says you agree to allow the staff of the hospital to provide medical care as directed by your physicians. There will also be a specific consent form for the operation, which details the specific procedure along with the more commonly recognized risks associated with that operation.

This consent form generally has a subsection that details your consent to receive blood or blood products if needed during the procedure. You can refuse blood transfusions and in most cases you'll still be able to have the surgery, but you should be aware that for this type of procedure, blood is given only in extreme life-or-death situations. Another form you'll be asked to sign is the consent for anesthesia. Many hospitals combine the operation consent and the anesthesia consent into a single document. It is very important that you read these forms and understand them. If you have questions, ask.

Robin's Story

I'm a nurse and while at my heaviest, I worked in a practice that handled diabetic patients. I was 266 at 5 feet, 4 inches and had Type 2 diabetes, high blood pressure, and severe rheumatoid arthritis. The doctor I worked for said that if I didn't get the weight off in five years, I'd be in a wheelchair. We had a patient come in for a follow-up who was heavy but had lost a lot of weight. I asked her how she did it, and she said she had a band.

My husband of 30 years thought I could lose the weight on my own, and he didn't want me to do the surgery. I found a band doctor, did the pre-op tests, then took out a second mortgage to get the band. Turns out my husband had issues at the beginning that I might find someone else if I lost weight. But when he went to the band doctor's seminar, he asked a lot of questions and was comfortable with the answers. So he got on board and now he's very supportive.

I got banded in February, and by the end of May I'd lost only 14 pounds. But I was taking Prednisone, a steroid that helps reduce inflammation to treat the arthritis. I knew the drug might affect my weight loss, but at that point I was starting to think I'd just thrown away thousands of dollars for nothing. When I got off the Prednisone, my weight started to drop.

Now, two and a half years out, my diabetes is under control, I'm decreasing the arthritis medication, and I feel great. I was taking two shots of insulin a day, and my blood sugar was over 300. And it was a cascade effect, because the Prednisone made my blood sugar problems worse. The lowest I got was to 189, but now I stay somewhere around 200 pounds. I dropped from a size 26 to a 14 and a half, I ride bikes, hike with my husband, and I feel so much better. I used to come home from work feeling exhausted. I feel I went from a nonproductive life to a productive one.

I've had some problems. At one point, I had my port flip. It turned completely upside down and had to be sewn back in. I've also had esophageal problems. My food sticks in my throat and holds there several seconds. They put me on a medication to help with the spasming. Mostly they blame the esophageal problems on the band. On fluoroscopy, you can see the fluid stop for several seconds, then drop down and go right through the band. I drink hot water in the morning before I take my pills to help. Cold things make the spasming worse. I heat my food, dry food bothers me, and I can't eat salads. I have to concentrate when I eat because if I phase out of what I'm doing and swallow too soon, I have problems. It's like I'm starting all over again with the band.

I've been cold since I lost weight, and I wasn't before. I use flannel sheets year round, wear warm pajamas when I didn't before, and I find myself snuggling in my quilts. Even in 100-degree weather I put on a sweater.

Also, my hair fell out about month four. It was thin and fine already, so I thought I was going to go bald. Now it's back to where it was, but for a while there I thought it wouldn't come back. And I'd like to get a tummy tuck or maybe a lower body lift because I do have that apron from the hanging stomach skin.

A friend and I decided to open our own clinic to do fills for patients banded in Mexico and to help diabetics patients. The band end is such a positive thing. We see people who are happy about losing weight, and it's so great. The diabetics whine a lot and are unhappy. We had a lady come in who had her leg amputated last year and her blood sugar was 300. I said to her, "I'll bet I know what you did. You had three donuts this morning." She said, "They should have a cure for this, and I should be able to eat whatever I want."

Sometimes I have that attitude as a band patient. I think I just want a french fry. I'm certainly not working at 100 percent. I know to get this last 30 pounds off I need to change my eating habits and increase my exercise.

It's interesting to work in a fill practice and see where the doctors put their ports. Mine is in the right lower abdomen and rubs against my clothes sometimes. Some put them on the left-hand side below the ribs in the waist area on the abdominal muscle. That can be a hard place to get to when patients are pretty fluffy, and we only use a 2-inch needle. We sometimes have these patients lift their head and their leg up. Some docs put them on the sternum between the breasts. Others put it right underneath the left breast on the lining of the ribs. A lot of women complain that their bras rub it at first, but it's really easy to access.

Part of our goal in our fill business is to help people pre-op make the best decision. We tell people they want to know what they're getting into. You don't want to jump into a decision. Some doctors don't have you do the liver-shrinking pre-op diet, and they have to lift the liver out of the way. One patient we had didn't do the pre-op diet, and his liver was so huge they had to open him up 6 inches and the doctor had to use his hand to hold the liver out of the way.

I'd like to see the pre-op liver-shrinking diet be a requirement for every band patient. It's my opinion that if you can't do the liver-shrinking diet, you're not going to make it as a bandster, because this is a lifestyle change.

We have a support group for band patients and bring in guest speakers. We had a chiropractor who talked about getting your center of balance back. He said that obese people walk back; they tip back to keep their balance. So when you lose weight, your body is out of balance. An exercise ball helps, and so does standing on one foot and closing your eyes, then doing the same thing on the other foot. He said that he removed the chairs from his classroom and introduced the exercise balls, and his students started experiencing better balance. I remember when I lost 50 pounds, my tail bone hurt when I sat, and I had to sit on a pillow for about four months. And I noticed the weight loss changed my balance.

What I've noticed is you have to take the parts of the program that work for you and let the rest go. There are times when I can't eat solid food. I know I should eat an egg for breakfast, but even the oatmeal sticks. So occasionally I do a protein shake for breakfast. Not everyone can even eat breakfast, but most people can eat lunch. I find for lunch I use a George Foreman grill a lot, and the meat is really moist.

I believe a lot of my weight issues have to do with what happened to me as a child. I lost my parents and had to live with my abusive brother-in-law. My siblings and I became his servants. I was the babysitter, housekeeper, and was abused all the time. I've had to work through issues around that.

With a lot of band patients, I see them get angry at society when they get thinner. I hear them say, "Why do people treat me well now when they didn't when I was fat? I'm the same person." I believe it works better if we let go of what people think. That's what I've done.

I have a son who is 23 years old and was 413 pounds at 6 feet, 4.5 inches. He was getting more and more depressed about his weight. So we took him to Mexico for a band. He's lost 100 pounds in a year with no fill at all. My husband is very supportive of him as well.

As for the changes in me, I think people listen to me more now that I'm not as heavy. It's hard to tell someone they need to watch their eating when you're heavy yourself. I was not a role model. When I decided to tell people I'd had the surgery, I had doctors all over the area sending patients to talk to me about the band. As a consequence of both my weight loss and my willingness to help others, I think I'm more respected.

The Day of Surgery

All the anticipation has led up to the day of surgery. This is typically a very exciting day for most patients. You should arrive at least an hour if not two hours prior to your scheduled procedure for a couple of reasons. First, you need some time to relax and get comfortable. If you are rushed or overly anxious, your blood pressure and your heart rate can go up, potentially complicating your anesthesia. Surgery is too important for you to be rushed. Besides, on the day of surgery, what else do you have to do that is more important? Having said that, I'm reminded of a lady several years ago who showed up five minutes before her scheduled surgery. When I asked her why she was late, she informed me that she had a standing appointment to have her hair done on that particular day, and nothing else was more important. I guess it's harder to get a hair appointment than it is to schedule surgery. I will say her hair did look nice!

Second, it is possible that if another procedure scheduled ahead of yours cancels, or takes less time than anticipated, the time of your procedure could be moved up. You want to be ready to go in case that happens.

Once you arrive at the hospital you'll be asked to change into a hospital gown, and the nurse will start an IV to begin giving you some fluids. You will also receive some IV antibiotics and a small injection of an anticoagulant, or blood thinner, called heparin. The antibiotic is given to help prevent infection, while the anticoagulant helps prevent blood clots.

While you are under anesthesia, blood will have a tendency to pool in the larger veins in your legs and pelvis. That is particularly true in patients who are extremely overweight. Blood that remains stagnant, even inside your own veins, will tend to clot, a condition known as venous thrombosis. If a clot forms it can block the flow of blood and lead to pain and swelling of the legs, ankles, and feet. More important, if this clotted blood breaks away from the wall of the vein, it will quickly travel back to the heart and be pumped up into the lungs. That is called a pulmonary embolus and is potentially a life-threatening situation, depending on the size and number of clots.

Pulmonary embolus is one of the most serious complications that can occur as a result of any bariatric operation, and the best treatment is prevention. So in addition to receiving heparin you will also be asked to put on a pair of elastic stockings to help keep the blood in your legs moving. As an added precaution, before the operation your legs will be wrapped with inflatable leggings called sequential compression devices, or SCDs, that will periodically massage your legs to promote normal circulation. You will need to continue to wear these stockings and SCDs until such time as you are up and about normally.

During your discussion with the anesthesiologist and the nursing staff, you will be asked many of the same questions that you've answered in the surgeon's office. While it may seem ridiculous to have to repeat the same information over and over again, this built-in redundancy is actually designed to help protect you from potential medical errors. There have been several highly publicized cases in which a patient got the wrong operation or received medications that were harmful, and everyone is acutely aware of these risks.

All the people who are involved in your care are charged with being on the lookout for potential problems, such as drug allergies, medication errors, and even getting you mixed up with another patient. While repeatedly being asked the same questions may make it seem like the staff and doctors are not communicating, the fact is that the more times you are asked about these things the safer you are. In fact, as a final step in that safety process, once you are in the operating room, but before the procedure is started, all the members of the surgical team stop what they are doing and have a "time-out." Everyone must agree on the identity of the patient, the procedure to be performed, and any drug allergies or other unusual circumstances about the case before proceeding.

Cynthia's Story

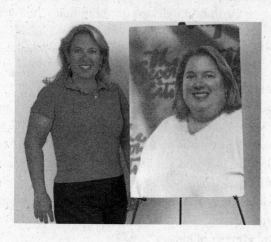

Cynthia, seven and a half years post-op at 145, shown with a photo of herself, pre-op, at 340.

I was one of the early band patients in the United States. I was banded on March 29, 1999, as part of the second round of FDA trials for the *LAP-BAND®*. I live a day's drive from New Orleans, where they were doing the band surgeries as part of the trials. My starting weight was 340 pounds at 5 feet, 2 inches tall. I now vary between 140 and 145, and I'm an inch shorter, at 5 feet, 1 inch. I think there was padding in my feet, and so I lost some height.

I went back to New Orleans every couple of months, as part of the protocol. And I got a fill about every other time I went back. At first, I didn't want anyone to know I had a band because I was embarrassed. But I got over that pretty fast. Now I tell people that those who've gotten a band are doing something proactive with their lives.

I've had a good experience being banded, but my first band did slip. The circumstances behind the slip were I got engaged in 2005 to a man who had five children. I'd always been single, so it was a stressful time for me. Before the wedding, I was struggling. I'd had similar trouble after my father died. The pattern was that whenever I got nervous or upset, my band slipped over my esophagus instead of under my esophagus. So once or twice a year my doctor would take out the fluid, wait a couple of weeks, and put the fluid back in.

When I got engaged, it got worse. I was productive burping and throwing up. My meals just wouldn't stay down. I knew that something wasn't right. They did tests, found out my band had slipped, and my doctor took out all the fluid. I picked up 25 pounds—*bam*—just like that. My doctor said, Why don't we replace the band now, instead of waiting until two weeks before the wedding? In both cases, my insurance paid for the bands. I remember being one of the few during the FDA trials that did have insurance to cover the band.

At first I had the band that holds 4ccs of fluid and got it replaced with a much bigger 9cc band. I'm one of the few people who've had both bands.

What I notice about the difference between the larger and smaller bands is it took longer to get to the sweet spot with the larger band, meaning that I had to have more adjustments to find the fill amount that was perfect for me. Another difference between the two is I now have more warning about being full with the big band. I can be chewing a bite and know I can have one more bite and that'll be all I can eat. With the smaller band, I got no warning. I'd have a bite ready and realize I couldn't swallow it—that I was full. I find it's nice to have a little more warning about when I'll be full.

I always say you don't know what you don't know. Back when I got banded there was so much less information. So I decided to do something about that. I've been very active in the banding community, doing seminars with doctors and even at one point opened my own business for banding care that I later sold to a band doctor.

In working with band patients, one thing I noticed is sometimes they can be like Veruca Salt, the girl from the movie *Charlie and the Chocolate Factory*, who wanted everything "NOW!" The weight loss is slow, and it's slow for a reason. The best part of this is it works, and the weight won't ever come back. I did all the diets, and the weight always came back. I kept waiting, with the band, for the other shoe to drop, and it never did. I advise people to go ahead, shop for a doctor and start the process with the doctor you like the best while you're still deciding whether or not to do it. Because once you decide, you'll want it done yesterday.

As for advice for band patients, I'd say do your homework and know what you're getting into. The patients who think they're just going to wake up one day and have lost 100 pounds are the ones who have a hard time. There is a process, and there are rules to follow. Banding is a surgery in which patients keep coming back, and both doctors and patients have to make peace with that. One of the things a band patient would be wise to find out is, Are they ever going to see their doctor again after the surgery? Is there a dietitian available? How about a psychologist?

The biggest change came when I'd lost about 60 pounds. It was interesting to me that I could be as huge as I was, take up so much space, and still be invisible. But once people started to notice me, I found it daunting. My life changed so much, I asked to see my band doctor for a talk. He told me my symptoms were from pure stress. I remember thinking I was going crazy. He put me on antidepressants, and I stayed on them until I got to my goal weight. At that point, my doctor told me to go talk to my therapist, and she gave me the tools to deal with people starting to notice me. I found, working with band patients, that a lot of people start self-sabotaging if they're not ready for the changes that occur.

I found myself and a lot of other people spent our time being fun and happy to make up for being overweight. It was amazing to me to see the transformation in people who've lost weight. They were people who had to work so hard at being cute and fun. I'm amazed when I think about how much I had to worry about hygiene and about dressing, how I had to go to specialty shops for clothes, and I knew I didn't look appealing. So I had to be the best friend, the fun person, and I worked hard at not being depressed because of the weight. As I lost the weight, I noticed I didn't have to be the fun one and go the extra mile. I found working with band patients, it was really neat to watch people become who they really are.

The band is a whole life change. Take me, for example. I'm married now, and I don't have the same job. I had a job in the travel industry where I was a human doormat. As I got thinner, I decided to stop being that person. For example, I stopped accepting calls from clients in the middle of the night. I didn't lose any clients, but it was an adjustment for me and my coworkers when I started to say no. I found out saying no is okay. But it was a stressful process and one that took some adjustment.

I do think that having the band and the boost in self-esteem it gave me was a big part of attracting my husband. I met him through a band patient. I had some people ask me if I told him I was banded, but I made sure he knew. Some people who lose weight are like kids in a candy store with dating. I wasn't that way. I decided that if I knew someone well enough to take my clothes off with them, then I knew them well enough to tell them about my band.

I've had lots of plastic surgery. At one point they called me the plastic surgery poster child. My stomach hung down to my knees, and my insurance paid for the tummy tuck. I've also had a breast reduction, my arms done, thighs, my back around my bra area, and a couple of revisions. I also got a low-profile port because the other port stuck out.

I've had the band for seven and a half years. I lost 210 pounds originally and have gained back 10 overall. I'm healthy, and I'm within a healthy weight category. But if you go by the weight charts, I should be at 120. However, I got down to 127 at one point and was so gaunt that people were asking me if I was okay. I think because I carried around so much weight before, I tend to be more compact and denser than the average person, almost like a former weight lifter.

The best part of the band is that it's reversible. I remember initially, I thought, "I'll get the band removed after I've lost all the weight." Two weeks after my surgery, I completely changed my mind, and now I say, "They'll take it off over my dead body."

Anesthesia

When everything is ready, you will be rolled into the operating room on a stretcher. You may or may not remember this particular event because the anesthesiologist will likely give you some medication that not only relaxes you but also has an amnesic effect. You will still be awake and able to cooperate with the staff; you just won't be able to recall much of the experience afterward.

Once you're in the operating room, a number of electronic devices will be connected to you to monitor your heart rate and the level of oxygen in your blood. You will be given some oxygen to breathe through a plastic mask that is placed over your mouth and nose. This is to ensure that your blood is fully saturated with oxygen before the anesthesiologist puts you to sleep.

To enable the surgeon to perform the operation, you must not only be asleep and unable to feel anything but you must also be totally relaxed. To accomplish this the anesthesiologist gives three different types of medications: (1) a narcotic-type drug that dulls the pain sensing areas in your brain, (2) an anesthetic drug that causes you to go to sleep and to stay asleep, and (3) a muscle relaxant that paralyzes your muscles. These drugs are given through the IV you had inserted when you first arrived in the holding area.

The most difficult part of the anesthetic is what is called the induction process, and the most critical part of induction is placing the airway tube, called an endotracheal tube, through your vocal cords and into the windpipe, or trachea, to maintain breathing. A significant number of morbidly obese people are classified as difficult intubations, and in these cases the anesthesiologist must be prepared to use any of a number of techniques to establish and maintain the patient's airway. The sequence and dosages of the various anesthesia medications is critically important in this process, especially the paralyzing drugs. Once the paralyzing drugs have been given, you will not be able to breathe on your own, and the anesthesiologist will have to do the work of breathing for you.

I've been asked many times why it is necessary for the patient to be paralyzed. The answer is really quite simple. Even when you are completely asleep, your muscles still move involuntarily in response to any stimulation. Laparoscopic operations require the abdominal cavity to be inflated with gas. Without paralyzing the muscles, that would simply not be possible. The muscles would respond by contracting down against the inflation process, and the surgeon would have no space inside the abdomen in which to work.

In recent years there has been a considerable amount written and a lot more said about what patients actually experience during operations, including their being able to remember hearing conversations and even experiencing pain. There is no doubt that such things can occur, but they are quite rare. Most surgical patients have no recollection of anything that goes on during their operation. For those who do have some recall, it is usually in the form of being able to hear people talking around them. That is because hearing is generally the last sense that is blocked by anesthetic drugs.

You are probably wondering why they don't just give enough anesthesia to make sure that such things can't occur. Well, most of the time that is precisely what the anesthesiologist does, but all of these medications wear off over time, and not every patient's body processes these powerful drugs exactly the same.

The anesthesiologist must balance the effects of the medications with the needs of the patient, and at the same time avoid overdosing. The ideal situation is for the full effect of the drugs to be immediate, and then be completely gone at precisely the same time the surgeon finishes the operation. But not everyone responds exactly the same to each drug given. If more medication is given than what you need, you could be asleep considerably longer than necessary.

Once the operation is over you will be taken from the operating room to the recovery room. Interestingly, like many other things in medicine, its name has changed. It is more accurately called the post-anesthesia care unit, or PACU. Your arrival in the PACU signals the beginning of your postoperative recovery, which will be covered in the next chapter.

9

What to Expect after Surgery

Any transition serious enough to alter your definition of self,
will require not just small adjustments in your way of living
and thinking, but a full-on metamorphosis.
—Martha Beck, *O Magazine,* "Growing Wings," January 2004.

Following most surgical procedures, once you are in the recovery room/PACU it is fair to say that "the hard part is over." But with the AGB that is not the case. While the surgical procedure itself may be over, the operation simply marks the beginning of the real work of changing a lifetime of habits, behaviors, and thoughts that lead to your obesity. Nevertheless, getting past the operation is truly a milestone in your weight-loss journey.

Immediately after Surgery

The first hour or so after surgery is spent in the PACU, where you will be carefully monitored as the effects of the anesthesia drugs gradually wear off. You may not even remember being in the PACU. I have had many patients tell me that the first thing they recall is waking up in their hospital room. This is despite the fact that I spoke with them and they spoke with me a few minutes after their operation. Most anesthesia medications cause a drug-induced amnesia, which is not necessarily a bad thing.

It is almost comical at times to hear a patient ask a question about the operation and appear to hear and understand the answer, only to repeat the same question within a few seconds. Sometimes patients will repeat the same question over and over, with the exact same words and the same vocal tones. The next day they never recall having had any conversation and will once again ask the same question. But this time, only once.

For those who are awake and alert in the PACU, the two most common complaints are pain and nausea. Both of these can often be prevented by giving appropriate medications in advance. If they occur despite these efforts, additional medications are readily available.

Pain following laparoscopic surgery is generally not a major problem. The small incisions are not typically the source of major pain. The exception may be the site where the injection port is placed.

Because the port is sutured to the muscle layer, it may cause an occasional sharp pain in the area, especially with moving, deep breathing, or coughing. But these are important activities after surgery, so if the pain is bad enough that it is restricting movement, pain medication will be given.

Not surprisingly, operations performed directly on or around the stomach are often followed by nausea once the patient is awake. Likewise, retching or vomiting after this type of surgery is not a good thing. It is possible it might do some

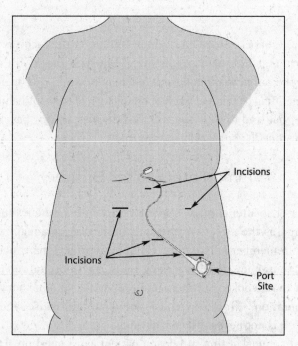

This figure shows the relative locations of the incisions and the location of the band, tubing, and port after the laparoscopic placement of the AGB.

serious damage, so it is very important to get nausea under control. The best way to deal with this problem is to give appropriate antinausea medications beforehand. For those patients who develop postoperative nausea, we have a wide variety of medications available. Fortunately this type of nausea is usually gone by the next day.

The Hospital Stay

Each patient remains in the PACU for an hour or so, or until they are awake and alert. They are then taken to a hospital room where they will stay until being discharged, usually the following morning. For the first few hours the nursing staff will be in and out of the room every hour or so checking blood pressures, making sure the IV is working properly, making sure the compression devices on your legs are working properly, and asking you about pain and nausea. Eventually, these visits become less frequent, allowing you some uninterrupted time to rest.

Many bariatric surgeons perform the AGB procedure on an outpatient basis, allowing patients to go home just a few hours after their operation. In many cases that practice is quite safe, but my own preference is to keep my patients in a hospital setting overnight. My rationale is that if patients are going to have problems after surgery, they are most likely to occur within that first 24-hour period. This includes serious issues such as heart attack, internal bleeding, or signs of stomach perforation. Granted, those may not be all that likely following an AGB operation, but morbidly obese patients are at higher risk for developing a variety of problems than patients of normal weight.

There is another reason I believe keeping patients in the hospital overnight is generally a good idea. Family members may or may not be comfortable providing even the basic care needs of someone following surgery. This can be a frightening job if you are not sure exactly what you should be looking for and what to do in the event you suspect a problem. Nurses are specifically trained not only to recognize potential problems but also to provide a calming environment. Patient and family alike can experience considerable anxiety when dealing with postoperative pain and nausea in the absence of professional help. Even just getting in and out of bed to go to the bathroom creates questions about what to do. All of these issues are much easier for everyone the next day than they are just six or eight hours immediately after surgery.

In addition to taking your vital signs and asking how you are doing, the nurse will also be encouraging you to breathe deeply and cough. This is extremely important because after surgery you will tend to take shallow breaths only, which can lead to retained secretions in your lungs, and eventually even cause pneumonia. To help improve lung function you will be encouraged to get out of bed and even take a walk in the hallway. Walking also improves the circulation in your legs and helps reduce the risk of blood clots.

A significant number of morbidly obese patients also suffer from sleep apnea. That is even more likely when you are under the influence of sedating medications. If you are one of those who require a positive pressure breathing machine to sleep, bring it with you to the hospital and use it as you normally would to sleep. Don't assume that the hospital will provide you with your CPAP or BiPAP treatment.

You will be connected to a monitoring device called a pulse oximeter, which is placed on your finger to measure the amount of oxygen in your blood. If your blood oxygen level is lower than normal, the nurse will place a small plastic tube in your nose or a mask over your face to supply you with more oxygen to breathe. You may also be hooked up to a heart monitor, particularly if you have a history of cardiac problems or an irregular heart beat.

If you have diabetes your blood sugars can fluctuate dramatically following surgery. The combination of not eating, receiving IV fluids, and the stress of surgery makes it difficult to predict exactly what your blood sugar will do. One thing is certain: your usual dosage of insulin or oral medication is not likely to be appropriate during this time. Instead, the nurse will check your blood glucose level every few hours so that the right amount of medication can be given.

To avoid getting dehydrated, you will remain on IV fluid until you are fully awake and able to take fluid by mouth. The continuous flow of fluids into your body will catch up with you, and eventually you will need to get up to the bathroom. Don't try to manage all the monitors and tubes by yourself. The nurse will need to help you for at least the first time or two.

Problems urinating are not common following obesity surgery, but occasionally patients are unable to urinate. This may be because of the effects of sedation or a pre-existing condition. If your bladder becomes distended and you can't void on your own, the nurse will need to insert a small tube, called a catheter, up into your bladder. Urinary difficulties of this kind are most often temporary, but if you continue to have trouble emptying your bladder it may be necessary to put in a catheter that remains in for an extended time. Fortunately, that is pretty rare following AGB surgery.

Between the IV, the blood pressure cuff, the compression devices on your legs, oxygen tubing, the oxygen monitor, the heart monitor, and the breathing machine you may feel like an astronaut, ready for take-off, or Gulliver trapped in the land of the Lilliputians. Just remind yourself that all this "stuff" is actually designed to help you get through your surgery safely.

Once you are awake, the nurse will offer you some ice chips or clear liquids to sip on. This will be the first time you will be swallowing anything after your band has been placed, so take it slow. Make sure you are sitting up, and take only small sips. If you try to swallow liquids while you are lying down flat, or nearly flat, the liquids may not want to go down. Even when sitting up you may get the feeling that there is something slowing down the passage of fluid into your stomach. That's the band.

Occasionally, patients describe some pain in their chest, back, or throat when they first start taking liquids, especially if the liquids are extremely hot or cold. This pain is due to a spasm in the lower esophagus that occurs as the esophagus is attempting to push the fluids past the resistance created by the band. The best way to avoid this problem is to drink very slowly and avoid hot or cold liquids. Carbonated drinks may also cause esophageal spasm, but the main problem they create is a feeling of being bloated. Once the gas gets below the band it can be very difficult to belch it back up, so it is best just to avoid sodas and sparkling water.

Checklist: Post-op Tips for Taking in Fluids

- ✓ Take small sips.
- ✓ Avoid hot or very cold liquids.
- ✓ Sit up when you swallow.
- ✓ Avoid carbonated drinks such as sodas or sparkling water.

Following surgery you will have some pain from the small incisions in your abdomen. Some patients describe their pain as severe, but most people describe it more as soreness rather than a real pain. Typically, they say it feels like they have just done a hundred sit-ups. To manage this postoperative pain, the nurse will give you medication either through the IV, as an injection, or as a liquid pain medication that is taken by mouth. The advantage of IV drugs is quick action, but they also tend to wear off more quickly. When drugs such as morphine or Demerol are given by injection into the muscle, they are a little slower to begin working, but they will generally last several hours. Oral medications are even slower to begin working, but are easier to take than a shot.

Postoperative nausea is also fairly common, and medication will be available to help control it. Generally the nausea will subside within a few hours, once the effects of the anesthesia wear off, but it is important to get the nausea under control and avoid vomiting. Antinausea medications are usually given either through the IV or as a rectal suppository. It doesn't make much sense to give someone who is nauseated any medication by mouth, since they are likely to bring it back up before it has a chance to take effect.

Some surgeons routinely require their patients to have a stomach X-ray the day after the band has been placed. This involves swallowing some liquid contrast material to see exactly where the band is in relation to the stomach and esophagus, and to make sure that there is no leakage. Others, and I include myself in this category, order this type of X-ray only in cases in which the operation was particularly difficult, or if the patient is having some problems swallowing.

Before you can go home from the hospital you will need to be able to take adequate fluids by mouth. On rare occasions, the band can create a complete blockage of the stomach. This may be due to excessive swelling of the stomach wall, or the band may have been too tight to begin with. Generally the passage through the band will open up over a two- or three-day period, but until it does you will need to remain in the hospital on IV fluids. It is extremely uncommon to have to take a patient back to surgery to remove or reposition the band, but that might be necessary if the obstruction persists.

Lorrie's Story

I heard about the band from a girlfriend in Las Vegas who asked me if I'd be interested in doing it with her. We called around to find the lowest price and discovered we could have it done for less in Mexico. When we went through the process to get the band, I just barely qualified. I'm 5 feet, 5 inches, and I started at 215.6 pounds. During the qualification process, my girlfriend backed out.

I've always been on the chubby side. But I could lose until I started menopause and quit smoking. After that, I could starve myself and not be able to lose the weight. Every year my aunt went on a water-only fast for 30 days early in the year. And I did that with her for a couple of years and lost 20 pounds in a month. I found that after the first week, you go through a period of headaches and being sick; then, after a week, you have all the energy in the world. But I'd gain the weight back. A friend of mine who is in the medical profession told me that when you get too overweight, your body is just not going to be able to lose. That's why you need something to help you.

I deal poker for a living and travel a lot. I figured if I had the surgery at the end of October, that'd give me the whole month of November to recuperate. I did the pre-op diet and had a talk with some of the doctor's staff before the surgery.

The easiest part of this process was doing the surgery. They kept me one night in the hospital, and the next night I went to a hotel. I went shopping, did a lot of walking, and none of it bothered me at all. Then I came home and sat around for a week and a half and didn't do anything strenuous at all. Just rested.

Just before I went back to work I had a massage by my regular massage therapist. The first week of working I had a lot of pain, and I wonder if it was because of the massage. On the table (when I'm dealing) I do a lot of stretching and moving. My port, my stomach, my back all hurt. I called the doctor's office, and they didn't think the massage was a problem. I took a lot of pain medication, and after about a week, the pain went away.

However, a friend of mine who had weight-loss surgery marvels at how fast I was up and around. He was almost 500 pounds, had the gastric bypass, and lost 240 pounds altogether. But he was laid up for months.

I just had my first fill at six weeks in Tijuana with the surgeon who did the band. Seven hours prior to the fill they asked me not to eat anything, just have water. And now I've been on yogurt, very liquid soups, Slimfast®, and water since the fill. I tried to eat an egg, and it wouldn't go down. They did tell me to go back to the post-op diet, meaning start back on liquids then to soft foods and then back to regular foods, since they expected I'd be a little swollen after the fill.

Since I travel a lot, wherever I go they have food and there's always room service. I think had I been home more, I probably could have gotten a good band diet going. But I really didn't have any idea what to eat. At times, I do feel kind of panicky. I tried a milkshake and could only get about a fourth of it down. It's uncomfortable to adjust to a fill.

I obviously have a fascination with food. But now people invite me out to dinner, and I don't always care to go. It used to be my whole social life was about where to eat. Now I'm planning what I'll do about Christmas dinner. I find I have more time, and I'm working more to keep myself busy. Early on, I had a couple of days where I didn't know what I should eat when I was in a casino. I went to the seafood buffet in Reno and it seemed like a waste, because I knew I was going to eat only four bites. I realize now my old pattern when I used to travel was I'd stop for breakfast, then get some Cheetos® to snack on in my car on the road. In fact, my car would be filled with food. Now all I get when I stop is water.

I consider the band a diet. It's the best diet I've ever been on, and it's going to work. It was so depressing before, when I'd diet, diet, diet—follow all the rules, get on the scale, and nothing. But with this, I do what they tell me and I get on the scale and I see results. I'm now down to 190 pounds, which is a loss of 25.4 pounds.

I love the band. I think it's the best thing anyone can do for themselves. I am encouraging my friends to do it.

Going Home

The vast majority of my patients are discharged from the hospital the morning after their band operation, but I don't allow them to drive themselves. The lingering effects of pain medications can alter judgment and reaction times for several days. You'll need to have someone drive you home, and it is probably wise to have someone stay with you for a day or two, until you are getting around comfortably and able to take care of yourself completely.

During those first few days at home you will probably take some of your pain medication that was prescribed by your surgeon. As long as you are taking pain medication it is potentially dangerous to be driving a car or operating heavy equipment or power tools. If you are otherwise feeling well, about 24 hours after your last prescription pain medication, it should be all right to drive yourself short distances.

Guidelines for Recuperating at Home

- Don't drive yourself home from the hospital.
- It's best to have someone stay with you for a couple of days after surgery.
- Driving is usually safe 24 hours after you've taken your last prescription pain medication and you're feeling well. The same goes for operating heavy machinery or power tools.
- Skin incisions need 48 hours to heal enough that water won't damage them. So wait two days to shower.
- Take it easy. Rest. Give yourself time to regain your strength.
- Don't remove the butterfly strips over your incisions. Let them fall off on their own, usually in a week to 10 days.
- Do walk, working up gradually to longer distances.

The first few days at home should be spent resting and recuperating from surgery. The physical stress of an operation is obvious, but having surgery can also be mentally and even emotionally draining. Give yourself some time to gain your strength before plowing back into your busy routine. It will pay major dividends in the long run and may even convince you that it's all right to slow down the pace of your life. After all, lifestyle change is precisely what you are trying to accomplish with the band, right?

One of the most common questions asked after surgery is "When can I take a shower?" I suggest to my patients that they wait until the second day after their operation. After about 48 hours the skin incisions are healed enough that water running across them will not be a problem. This means showers only for the first week. Soaking in a tub should be avoided for the first week, and longer if there is any persistent drainage from the small incision sites.

I typically close the incisions with a type of suture that is designed to dissolve, and all the sutures are under the skin. To help support these sutures, we place small sterile tapes or "butterfly" strips across each incision. Additional dressings are placed over the incisions, and these can be removed about the time you take your first shower. But leave the sterile tapes on until they begin to fall off by themselves, usually about a week to 10 days later.

While getting enough rest is important, you shouldn't just lie in bed all the time. That is a recipe for problems, including blood clots and pneumonia. You should be up and moving around frequently. If the weather is nice, get outside and walk around the neighborhood. The fresh air will do you good. Start out slowly, and gradually work your way up to walking greater distances. The sooner you get started walking, the sooner you'll gain your strength back.

My Words Give Me Back My Power
G. Dick Miller, Psychologist

Does it really matter what we call something? What words we use? If I say, "I need something to eat," and you say, "It would be in my best interest to have something to eat," aren't we saying essentially the same thing? My contention is we're not.

The words we use can and do make a difference. Here's why. Certain words imply I have no rational choice. If I'm saying, "I should," or "I need," or "I have to," I'm sending the message to myself and others that I have given up my right to choose. My message is that someone or something outside of me is forcing me to do something I don't want to do. And if I don't want to do it, eventually, I'll find a way not to. In other words, I can create malcontent and rebellion in myself that will eventually lead to my making harmful choices by simply using language that gives away my power.

If I say, "I can," "I want to," or "It would be in my best interest to," I give myself back my power both in my own eyes and with others. Then I choose. No one is making me. And if I have decided, I'm not going to be expending my time and energy finding a way out. I allow myself the freedom of choice and give myself back my power.

Should, can't, never, always, right, wrong—these are all absolute words that are not in our best interests to use. Use of them is very dishonest and manipulative. We use these words because we don't honestly believe we can attack a problem and solve it. We don't believe we can have an honest approach. We want a trick, a gimmick, because we don't trust that we can do, or will do, what's in our best interests.

Rational vs. Irrational Word Choices

Irrational (Implies No Choice)	Rational (Implies Choice or Alternative)
should	could, wish, best
need	want to, smart to
have to, got to	want to, in my best interest
can't	want not, choose not
never	seldom
always	usually, often
right	in my opinion, I agree with
wrong	in my opinion, I disagree with

So, yes, the terminology does matter. It matters a lot. For example, with head hunger, I can create a negative situation for myself if I'm not personally honest. If I call anxiety or stress "hunger," then it makes sense for me to treat it with food.

But if I can learn to identify my uncomfortable feeling, be honest with myself, and choose to call it what it is, anxiety or stress, then I have a whole range of choices. All of the options for treating anxiety become available to me once I correctly name my discomfort. And this change in my thinking allows me to make a better decision for myself.

What I call things has a domino effect in my thinking. I can make the domino effect work for me if I work to change my language around my choices.

Medication Needs

Obviously, your need to take pain and nausea medication should decrease rapidly as the incisions heal. Occasionally, I'll have a patient tell me that they are still taking prescription pain medications a week or more after surgery, but that is unusual. If you still feel the need to be taking pain killers after the first week it could signal that there is a problem, and you should make your surgeon aware of the situation. However, recognize that sometimes people just like the way their medications make them feel, and continue to use "pain" as the reason for taking dose after dose of these powerful medications. Addiction to narcotic pain relievers is a real risk for some people, especially if they have a prior history of similar behavior. So if your surgeon refuses to refill your pain medication prescription, it is probably in your best interest.

Checklist: Taking Medication Post-op

✓ Pain medication can become addictive. So your surgeon may not want to refill your postoperative pain medication after a certain point.

✓ For your regular medication, you will need to crush pills or open capsules and mix medication with juice or water. Before doing this, check with your prescribing physician and MAKE SURE THIS IS SAFE.

✓ There may be liquid alternatives for your medications available, so ask.

✓ If you are taking medication to lower your blood pressure, monitor your blood pressure carefully. Sometimes blood pressure drops dramatically post-op with band patients, and your regular doctor may need to adjust your medication downward or eliminate it altogether. Be especially aware of feeling weak or dizzy, as that may be a sign your blood pressure is getting too low.

✓ If you have diabetes, monitor your blood sugar levels carefully. Often band patients need to adjust insulin or other diabetes medications downward, so be sure to check your blood sugar before giving yourself shots or taking your medication.

Other medications you were taking before the operation will generally need to be resumed afterward. This can present a problem if the pills are large. Any pill or capsule could potentially get stuck in the narrowed area of the stomach created by the band. If possible you should crush your pills or open the capsules and mix the medication with juice or water to allow it to go down easily. But before you do that, you should contact the physician who prescribed the medication to make sure it is safe to do so. Your pharmacist will also be able to advise you as to whether it is safe to alter your pills in this way, or whether a liquid alternative is available.

For those patients with diabetes or high blood pressure, it is more important than ever to monitor blood sugar levels and blood pressure regularly. The dramatic change in your diet can greatly affect these measurements, which can then necessitate changes in your medication dosage. This is particularly true for patients with diabetes. For those who routinely use insulin, you can easily overdose if you resume your usual dosage without checking your blood glucose level frequently. Remember, you are not eating anywhere near the same number of calories that you did before, and your blood sugar will naturally be lower.

Blood pressure is often similarly influenced during the postoperative period. Many patients need to reduce their blood pressure medications long before a significant amount of weight has been lost. It's important to check your pressure frequently, especially if you begin to feel weak or dizzy. If your pressure becomes lower than anticipated, you should contact your physician and let him or her adjust your medicines.

Returning to Normal Activity

After surgery you will also need to return gradually to your normal physical activities and start getting some exercise. This needs to begin soon after you get home, with walking, but you should limit any lifting to a maximum of 10 pounds for the first 10 days. After that the limit can be raised to 20 pounds for the next 20 days. So, after about a month you should be able to lift any amount you were able to lift prior to the surgery.

A number of patients participate in water aerobics and are eager to get back to that activity, which is great. However, waiting a week or so will allow the incisions time to heal enough to make it safe to be in the pool.

The big question is always "What about work?" If you have a desk job, or one that does not include much physical activity, you may be able to return to work within just a few days. For patients with more physically demanding jobs, it is usually necessary to stay off work for a couple of weeks. But this can vary, depending on the patient's general health, how rapidly they are recovering, the type of work they do, and other individual circumstances. The decision is ultimately up to the surgeon.

As you know by now, the whole idea of placing a band around your stomach is to restrict your food intake. The problem is that the degree of restriction changes over time following placement of the band. Initially the stomach is bunched up inside the band, creating a relatively small opening for food to pass through. That is why initially only liquids will pass through the band.

However, over the next few weeks the wall of the stomach gradually stretches out, remodeling itself around the band, creating a larger opening so food can pass through.

*Recommended Postoperative Diet**

Days 1–2   Clear liquids (32–64 ounces per day).

Day 2   Add protein drink (40–70 grams per day).

You'll find recipes for protein shakes on pages 144–145.

Days 3–4   Add full liquids, V-8 juice, thin cream soups, and yogurt.

Days 5–6   Add applesauce, pudding, smoothies, and banana.

Days 7–8   Add mashed potatoes, cream of wheat, and (baby food–style) well-cooked vegetables, vegetable soup, and legumes (beans) that have been well cooked (no grits, rice, pasta, or peanut butter).

Days 9–10   Add baked potato, oatmeal, soft boiled and scrambled eggs, cottage cheese, and canned pears (try adding low-fat cheese to eggs and potatoes).

Days 11–12   Slowly add fresh fruits; chew well and eat slowly; continue protein supplement drink, 64 oz. per day.

Days 13–15   SLOWLY add baked fish, tuna (with fat-free mayonnaise), toast or crackers, small amounts of rice, pasta, vegetables (except asparagus, celery, and corn), and whole-grain cereal (granola bars, protein bars).

Days 16–28   You're ready to try baked turkey and chicken and salads. Try one new food at a time, in small (1–2 oz.) servings, and chew, chew, chew.

Days 29–56   You can move on to ground beef, then gradually add roast beef, ham, and sausage. Steak should be last, and beef may always be problem. Bread may also be a problem no matter how well you chew it.

As the opening enlarges, fluids and even solid food will begin to pass through more easily. That doesn't mean that two weeks following surgery you will be able to eat a steak dinner. Some patients have more restriction than others post-op, but for most, they are pretty restricted in the beginning and there's a gradual change to less restriction. So to accommodate this changing level of restriction, we place patients on a progressive diet for the first few weeks. It starts with liquids, and then various solid foods are added as the opening enlarges. I've included the table (page 126) we give postoperative patients that gives our specific instructions for reintroducing foods.

Different programs will likely have different recommendations as to what you can and cannot eat in the postoperative period. Some may be fairly regimented like ours, while other may be much less specific. The important thing for you to realize is that the apparent tightness of the band will decrease significantly during the first few weeks, allowing you to eat more. Eventually, if you don't have the band tightened, filled, adjusted, or whatever they call the process in your doctor's practice, the band simply will not work.

DAYS 1 and 2	DAY 2	DAYS 3 and 4
Clear liquids Broth, gelatin, juice, popsicle No Straws!	Add supplemental protein drink, such as protein shakes 3–4 scoops protein powder/day, 24 grams per scoop Add chewable adult multivitamin and calcium daily as recommended	Add full liquids, V-8 juice, thin strained cream soups, and smooth yogurt 3–4 scoops protein powder/day, 24 grams per scoop
DAYS 5 and 6	**DAY 7**	**DAYS 8–10**
Add apple sauce, sugar-free pudding, smoothies and banana 3–4 scoops protein powder/day, 24 grams per scoop	Add baked potato (no skin), oatmeal (preferably unsweetened), egg substitute preferably, soft boiled and scrambled eggs, cottage cheese and canned pears (try adding low-fat cheese to eggs and potatoes) 3–4 scoops protein powder/day, 24 grams per scoop	Add mashed potatoes, "light" or fat-free margarine, salad dressings, sour cream, etc.; cream of wheat, and baby food Add well-cooked vegetables, vegetable soup, and well-cooked legumes (beans) 3–4 scoops protein powder/day, 24 grams per scoop
DAYS 11 and 12	**DAYS 13–15**	**DAYS 16–28**
Slowly add fresh fruits (no skin) Chew well Eat slowly Continue 3–4 scoops protein powder/day, 24 grams per scoop	SLOWLY add baked fish, tuna (with "fat-free" mayonnaise), toast or crackers, small amount of rice, pasta, vegetables (except asparagus, celery, and corn) and whole grain cereal (granola bars, protein bars) 3–4 scoops protein powder/day, 24 grams per scoop	STOP PROTEIN DRINKS or SHAKES You'll be ready to try baked, skinless turkey, chicken, lean ground beef, and salads
DAYS 29–56	**Dr. Sewell's Golden Rules**	**Goals**
Gradually add roast beef and lean pork Steak should be last!	Eat until comfortable, NOT FULL. Choose protein first, eat slowly, chew well. Drink liquids 15 minutes before or 2 hours after meals. Liquids will not satisfy hunger. Exercise daily.	Set daily protein and fluid intake goals. Determine your protein and fluid intake requirements with your doctor, dietitian, or at FitDay.com.

This detailed guide for introducing foods is given to each of my postoperative band patients. It is provided courtesy of the MASTER CENTER® for Minimally Invasive Surgery—Texas, LLP.

And now that you're starting your new life with the AGB, here are the golden rules for success. It will take a certain amount of experimentation to learn to follow these golden rules. I'll cover them in more detail later, but let me introduce them to you here. (There is also a list of 10 rules distributed by a band manufacturer on page 131.)

Checklist: Dr. Sewell's Golden Rules for AGB Patients

✓ Eat until you are comfortable, NOT FULL!
✓ Choose protein first—you need 50 to 70 grams of protein per day.
✓ Eat slowly and chew your food well.
✓ Don't drink 15 minutes before or during meals and for two hours after eating.
✓ Liquids will not satisfy your hunger, so you need to eat something.
✓ Exercise daily.

Conclusion

So far we've covered what to expect physically before and after surgery, but we haven't really addressed one of the most important aspects of the AGB process: adjusting the band. Following surgery, most patients begin to experience weight loss, but as they adapt to the band and the postoperative swelling subsides, their weight loss slows significantly. The most unique feature of the AGB is its adjustability. This is the topic of the next chapter.

10

Adjustments (Fills) and Eating Strategies

Always bear in mind that your own resolution
to succeed is more important than any one thing.
—Abraham Lincoln

Once you have a band you need to learn how to make it work for you in your effort to develop your new lifestyle. Adjustments to the band (known as fills) will help, but they must be combined with a learning process to change the way you eat. This process is critical to your successful weight loss and is the focus of this chapter.

The First Few Weeks Post-op

The first few weeks following placement of the band are unique because you're not likely to repeat them, and they are usually fairly structured. Our patients are provided a postoperative diet to follow. While the diet may seem stringent, most people are unaware that their stomach moves continuously as they digest food. So we encourage patients to carefully follow the reintroduction of foods listed in Chapter 9 so as to create as little stress as possible on the sutures during the healing process. We've found that at least for the first few weeks, almost everyone is all smiles because they are not hungry and continue to lose weight.

There are a few patients who after surgery do not experience restriction in their ability to eat, or those who experience total restriction for a few days post-op. Frankly, while it may be uncomfortable or frustrating to be in one of the extremes, it doesn't matter long term. The course of action is the same. You and your body must grow accustomed to the band, and the band eventually has to be adjusted to suit your unique requirements. In addition, you face the task of learning a new lifestyle and new strategies for eating.

As I have mentioned, the norm is that post-op patients don't experience hunger at all, and are usually very restricted in their ability to eat. Most have to stay on liquids in the beginning and gradually graduate to solid foods. While it may be hard to believe when you first get the band, after a few weeks the tightness of the band decreases significantly. The functional opening typically enlarges enough that in six weeks or so patients are able to eat nearly the same as they did before surgery. That is because the wall of the stomach remodels itself by stretching and thinning out under the band. Eventually the size of the banded opening becomes about the same size as the esophagus, and virtually anything that can be swallowed will pass through the band.

There is usually fat between the stomach and the band. The removal of this fat during surgery is not attempted, because it's dangerous and lengthens the surgery. And the body will naturally metabolize the fat as it uses up these extra energy stores over time. However, the fat does affect the shape of the opening, and that can become significant in the fill process, as you'll see later in the chapter.

As the stomach opening returns to normal, patients also notice a gradual return of hunger between meals. It's at this point that many will come into the office complaining, "This thing isn't working. Are you sure you put a band in there?" We expect patients to experience hunger the way they did preoperatively. While this can be cause for alarm to someone who may be, for the first time, experiencing some control over hunger, we see it as a sign the healing process is progressing normally.

Most surgeons wait until about six weeks after the surgery to perform the first adjustment to the band. If an adjustment is done earlier, there is risk of actually creating an obstruction. Six weeks seems to be a reasonable time to wait, but I have to admit that I have adjusted a few patients in the four- to five-week period. I've had others that seemed to be doing very well losing weight with no adjustment, so I've waited several months before tightening their bands.

Up to this point, the process is more or less the same for each band patient. But when it comes to adjusting the band, every patient is different. In part this is due to variations in anatomy. As I have already mentioned, some people have a large amount of fat around the stomach, which causes the band to be more restrictive.

But even more important is the fact that each patient tends to change their behavior at a different rate. The same size opening in the band may feel very tight for someone who is still eating too fast, taking large bites, and not chewing adequately. In comparison, someone who has begun to make more progress to change their eating behaviors will find the same opening less restrictive. So the process of tightening the band must be individualized to meet the needs of each patient.

Ten Rules for Eating with the Adjustable Gastric Band*

1. Eat slowly and chew thoroughly (approximately 15 to 20 times a bite).
2. Eat only three small meals a day.
3. Stop eating as soon as you feel full.
4. Do not drink while you are eating.
5. Do not eat between meals.
6. Eat only fresh food.
7. Avoid fibrous food.
8. Drink enough fluids during the day.
9. Drink only low-calorie liquids.
10. Exercise at least 30 minutes a day.

From the LAP-BAND® brochure distributed by BioEnterics Corporation, 2000

How Adjustments (or Fills) Are Accomplished

It is clear that simply placing a band around the stomach has limited effectiveness, because the stomach wall adapts to a static restriction. The beauty of the AGB is its flexibility. The tightness can be modified for a custom fit to suit each individual's needs. This process is called getting an "adjustment" or a "fill," meaning that saline is added to the band to contract the size of the opening.

The adjustment procedure is actually very simple. A special needle is used to inject a solution of sterile saline into the port, which was placed under the skin as part of the surgery. At that time, the port and the band tubing were filled with saline before they were implanted, so that when the patient has their first fill, and the fluid is injected into the port, it causes the balloon inside the band to inflate. The enlarging balloon acts like a tourniquet around the stomach, narrowing the opening between the small upper stomach pouch and the rest of the stomach.

As part of the adjustment process, the skin over the port is cleaned with an antiseptic solution, and then a small amount of local anesthetic is injected into the skin to numb the area. A larger, specialized needle is then inserted through the skin and through the silicone portion of the port. Saline solution is then injected into the system.

The needle used to adjust the band is designed specifically to pass through the silicone part of the port without damaging it. If someone were to use a typical hypodermic needle, like the ones used to give you an antibiotic shot into muscle, that needle would actually remove a small core of silicone, which would leave a hole where the saline would eventually leak out. If the saline leaks out, the band becomes loose and ineffective. That is the single most important reason you should never have the band adjusted by anyone who is not thoroughly familiar with the process and has the appropriate equipment.

The Band Is Not a Magic Bullet
Jessica Walker, Dietitian, M.S., R.D., L.D.

I've been working with band patients for several years now in the role of helping them with nutritional counseling. What I've learned is that the band is not a magic bullet. I didn't think it would be, but the more experience I get the more I see that the band as a tool works very well for weight loss.

Most people are pretty enthused in the beginning, because they lose with almost anything they do simply because they're taking in fewer calories no matter what they're eating. But as time goes on, the weight loss slows or stalls when people fall back into old habits, such as poor food choices, drinking with meals, and the like. Most people don't continue to lose because they're taking in too many calories, which may indicate that they need a fill. But I do see people on occasion who are not losing because they take in too few calories. One woman was eating only vegetables and dried cereal, which amounted to between 500 and 600 calories a day. She wasn't losing. Her body was hanging on to the fat. I tried to figure out a way she could add protein through beans or some meat, so she could up her calorie count and get her body back to using up those fat stores.

There are plenty of ways around the band, and people find them. From my experience, if patients cannot figure out the main issue or issues they have that caused food problems to begin with, the band won't help them. Usually I'm the last resort for those people. Out of the hundreds of successful patients in our band program, I often see the small percentage who haven't lost much after two years or who are back up to where they started; they are in my office desperate to figure out why.

In a nutshell, my experience is that people have problems when they move away from the band eating guidelines. The most successful patients are the ones who avail themselves of the monthly support group. Those folks are often self-correcting by taking a look at what they're doing and not doing as they listen to other band patients share their experiences. And in almost every case in which band patients are stalled with their weight loss, they identify a band guideline or two they've either not followed or gotten away from.

We see people needing fills periodically during their band journey. I've seen the surgery, and it's amazing how much fat is packed between the organs and around the stomach that the surgical team has to work around to place the band. So while people talk about how their band has loosened up, it's not actually the band that has changed, it's everything around it. One of the clues there's been a change and a fill is needed is that patients notice they can eat more. So we encourage them at that point to come in for a fill.

We don't encourage calorie counting. But what I've seen is when people get frustrated about their weight loss they go back to a lot of old diet practices such as calorie counting. Band patients are better off eating solid foods, but they often go to oatmeal or yogurt, both of which are good, nutritious foods, but not foods that will stick with you from one meal to the next. Sometimes you have to shift your mindset. We encourage people to stop worrying about calories, have something you want since you'll have only a couple of bites, but make sure that overall you're making good, solid food choices, such as getting the necessary protein.

We have speakers come to the support group and talk about topics of interest to patients, such as plastic surgery or new information on exercise. Daily exercise is important. People often get to where they don't want to be without it.

Sleep is also an important issue, since obesity and lack of sleep are linked. We are having someone come from the sleep disorders center to talk to our latest support group meeting. We often see that people who work third shifts or who have trouble sleeping also have trouble with their weight. One reason is that the body doesn't work correctly without enough sleep. But the other, more probable reason for weight gain in sleep-deprived people is that they're often looking for a pick-me-up. No one reaches for a vegetable or a piece of fruit when they're tired—they reach for high-calorie foods and usually foods that are sweet.

Another thing I see a lot is that people have a list of 30 foods they can't eat. I encourage people to make note of a food they don't tolerate, eliminate the food for now, but try a small amount again in a week or two. Sometimes people find out that they can tolerate a food but they took too big a bite the first time or they didn't chew it enough. In other words, they find out the problem wasn't the food at all. There might, however, be just a couple of foods that always give you trouble.

Finally, I've seen hundreds and hundreds of people get the band, but I've not once seen anyone say, "I wish I'd never gotten this band." That is true even with people who didn't lose as much as they thought, or with people who gained a little back. And while I've seen published statistics that say people stop losing after two years, I'm seeing people continue to lose past two years out. And I think that's great.

How Much Fill Do You Need?

The key to making the band a useful weight-loss tool is to create restriction without obstruction. If the band is too tight the patient may have trouble even swallowing liquids. If it is too loose, the patient will be able to eat too much. So, what is the right amount? Frankly, each patient is different. Should you have one major adjustment or multiple small adjustments? These are matters of considerable debate, even among surgeons who do this every day. Compelling arguments can be made to support a variety of adjustment styles.

Some surgeons suggest that the best way to adjust the band is to tighten it to a specific, predetermined size. To do so requires the use of fluoroscopy to watch the adjustment process while the patient swallows X-ray contrast material. The contrast material can actually be seen passing through the banded opening. The amount of fluid in the band is then precisely adjusted to create the desired size opening. This type of adjustment is considerably more expensive to perform because of the use of fluoroscopy; sometimes it is spoken of in shorthand as an "adjustment under fluoro." Also, since the procedure involves X-ray imaging, many surgeons have the adjustment performed by a radiologist rather than doing it themselves.

The drawback to using fluoroscopy, in which the band is tightened all at once, is that most patients experience considerable trouble eating. In other words, they are forced to make major changes in their eating habits without any preparation. When you've been eating a particular way for many years, it isn't easy just to suddenly slow down, take small bites, and stop when you are full. Old habits, and in particular the automatic process of eating, die very hard. Even the most highly motivated patients often find it difficult to cope with a sudden and major change in how they feel every time they try to eat.

One method that some patients employ to deal with this sudden problem is to resort back to a liquid diet. Obviously, though, that defeats the whole purpose of the band. But when patients feel as though they are starving, and everything they eat comes back up, they will eat whatever they can keep down. This includes high-calorie creamed soups, ice cream, chocolate, and other liquids. Not surprisingly this can lead to failure to lose weigh, protein deficiency, and even depression.

Certainly not everyone struggles to the point of having to resort to a liquid diet, but some do. An alternative style for adjusting the band involves multiple smaller saline injections over a period of time. These adjustments are typically performed in the surgeon's office and do not require fluoroscopy. By adding fluid to the band gradually over several weeks or even months, the patient is able to change their eating habits in smaller steps. It usually takes several adjustments of this type to reach the same level of tightness that is achieved with one fluoroscopic adjustment. However, patients spend less time spitting up and are somewhat less likely to resort to high-calorie liquid foods. But the down side is that early on, patients are still able to eat relatively normally, so their weight loss is often somewhat slower than anticipated.

Either approach to adjusting the band can be used effectively, provided that patients are instructed as to what they should expect. Personally, I prefer the gradual method, with adjustments being made no more often than every two or three weeks. I typically start out with an initial adjustment of 1.5 milliliters for patients with a standard 4 ml band, or 5 milliliters if they have one of the larger bands. After each adjustment the patient comes back into the office in two weeks to be weighed. At that time they meet with the dietitian to discuss their changing eating behaviors. If their weight begins to plateau, or if they are not feeling much restriction, I'll add 0.2 to 0.3 milliliters if it is a standard band, or 0.5 to 1.0 milliliters if it is a larger band.

It is surprising how sensitive some patients are to even minor adjustments to their band. It is possible to go from feeling only minimal restriction to being unable to keep anything down with only a small change in the volume of fluid in the band. Immediately following each adjustment I have each patient swallow 1 or 2 ounces of liquid, just to make sure they are still able to swallow. Despite passing this ritual, every once in a while I'll have a patient return within 24 to 48 hours complaining that they just can't keep anything down, and I'll have to take some of the fluid out.

The band, the tubing, and the port compose a closed system, so once fluid is injected into this system it remains there until it is removed. However, sometimes a small amount of air can become trapped in the port or in the tubing, taking up a small amount of space. During the initial adjustment, as fluid is added to the system, this air is flushed out into the balloon portion of the band. Here the Silastic membrane allows the air to leak slowly out of the system. The result is a gradual loss of restriction, and patients come in a few weeks later with the story that they felt much tighter right after the adjustment, but then it seemed to get loose again. When another adjustment is performed the amount of fluid in the band is less than expected. When that happens, it was not the saline that leaked out, only the air.

Joyce's Story

I've been overweight ever since I was a five-year-old kid. At age 16 I went to a diet doctor, did the pills and the shots, and got down to a size 9. I remember eating everything and still lost weight. Back then it took me a year to take off the weight, but I couldn't stay on the pills forever. Once I went off, it took only six months to put the weight back on.

When I had gallbladder surgery two years ago, at 4 feet, 11 inches and 250 pounds, I was too big for the surgeon to do it laparoscopically. Afterward, my doctor told my brother and my family I'd never see 80, even though my mom had just turned 80. I'm 56.

I had a lot of problems, such as blood pressure issues, cholesterol, and diabetes. Diabetes runs in my family, so it was a foregone conclusion I'd have it.

I'd read about the band, saw Dr. Sewell, and decided to have the surgery in April of 2005. I started at 241 pounds, with a BMI of 48. Back before the surgery, I went to the store and couldn't get halfway through, I was so tired. I'd waddle instead of walk.

Now at about a year and a half out, I'm down 61 pounds to 180 and my BMI is 36.4.

My biggest challenge is bread. I can eat it, but it's rough, so I stay away from it, even though I miss it a lot. I also stay away from sodas, when before I'd have six to eight of them a day. Pasta works for me, but I sometimes have a hard time with eggs.

I have not been as strict on myself as I probably should be. I figure it took me all this time to get this weight on, so if it takes me some time to get it off, then that's okay. As a consequence, I haven't watched everything I eat.

In addition, I've increased my exercise. I go to a fitness center where I walk on the treadmill and do water aerobics. Exercise makes me feel better. And I notice a big change in my energy level. I've been doing ballroom dancing for about 30 years, and I can do a lot more now and enjoy it more. Before I'd do two or three dances and I'd be pooped. Now I can dance the whole evening. I will have to start looking for some new gowns, though, because my old ones are getting too big.

I'm still taking medication for Type 2 diabetes, but my blood pressure has gone down quite a bit and I think I'll be off that medication soon.

I will be paying on the surgery for 10 years, but I have no regrets about doing this. I have to consider myself lucky, as a lot of people who get the band have to do it completely on their own. My insurance at least paid part of it. I do notice significant savings on what I used to spend on food and clothing, especially since I've gone from a size 22 to a size 16.

There have been a few issues. At one point I thought my port might have a leak, because I was restricted after my last fill then suddenly I didn't feel any restriction. When he checked the fill, I was supposed to have 3.3ccs and I had only 3.0. He filled it again, then asked me to come back and be checked in a couple of weeks. When I went back, I still had restriction and the fill was at 3.3ccs, so there was no leak. If there had been a leak, it would require day-surgery in which Dr. Sewell would take out the old port and put in a new one.

My port has moved since I lost weight. It's at my waistband now. Since I have a sitting job, the placement of the port is sometimes an issue, and I've talked to Dr. Sewell about moving it.

If I had any advice to someone considering a band, it would be to go for it. Personally, I wouldn't have considered the gastric bypass because I think it's too dangerous. There's danger in anything you do, but the risk was too high for me. With the band, I was comfortable with the risk. And I've heard too many stories about gastric bypass patients gaining their weight back, and some bypass patients are even going for the band on top of their bypass.

I would also recommend a support group of some kind. I signed up for the two-year support plan with the psychologist in Dr. Sewell's program. I am part of an online group, and I also go to Dr. Sewell's band support group meetings. I find the live support group very helpful, and I really enjoy it a lot.

Can You Lose Your "Sweet Spot"?

Once the proper amount of restriction is obtained, the so-called sweet spot, most patients lose between 1 and 2 pounds each week and everything is as it should be—right? Well, not exactly. Things inside the body have a habit of changing. It is quite common for patients to go along very well for several months after getting just the right amount of fluid in their band, but then gradually the band seems to be less restrictive. This may be in part caused by a gradual thinning of the stomach wall. However, the most logical explanation is that the fatty tissue that occurs naturally around the upper part of the stomach and is actually inside the band is decreasing as the patient loses weight. As this fat disappears it allows the stomach channel to enlarge, even though the amount of fluid in the band has remained unchanged. This explains why additional minor adjustments to the band may be needed every now and then until the patient's weight stabilizes.

It has been interesting for me to observe how many patients tend to become obsessed with the exact amount of fluid in their band. This may be a product of the nearly continuous discussions that go on between band patients, each one comparing every aspect of their situation with the experience of other patients. There are numerous Internet chat sites where band patients describe in detail the exact volume that they have in their band, as well as how much they think they should have, how much their friend has, and so on. But, as I stated earlier, every patient is different. An amount that seems to be just right for one patient may not provide anything close to the proper restriction for another.

After several years of doing adjustments I have discovered an unanticipated problem with the multiple adjustment approach. I refer to it as "adjustment addiction," and it is somewhat difficult to describe. Obviously, some patients who suffer from morbid obesity also have truly addictive personalities. Virtually anything and everything they get involved with has the potential to become an addiction. This can even include band adjustments. Despite doing quite well, losing a pound or two a week, these patients believe that continually adjusting the band helps to ensure their continued success. I believe that these patients are not so much craving another "needle stick," but instead are simply insecure in their own success. Generally these patients have not yet accepted the fact that it is their behavior, not the band, that is causing them to lose weight.

In many instances, individuals with addictive personalities don't recognize their own behaviors as addictions and invariably deny it when confronted. That is the source of potential conflict between the patient and the team of professionals attempting to deal with this situation. The easiest thing for the surgeon to do is provide another fill. Put a little in—take a little out—the process can become an endless quest, searching repeatedly for just the right amount of fluid in the band. In this situation the surgeon actually becomes the "adjustment addiction" enabler.

Reversing the patient's fixation on the band and their "need" for an adjustment requires recognizing the problem, and then approaching the patient honestly with positive reinforcement. Everyone within the comprehensive program—the surgeon, the dietitian, the exercise physiologist, the psychologist, and the supporting staff members—must recognize the situation and provide the patient with a consistent, positive message, emphasizing the patient's role in their own success.

Another problem I see is other patients who come in for regular adjustments but never seem to achieve the weight-loss success they expected. Typically these are individuals who expected the band to do all the work for them. By getting another adjustment they hope to lose weight and avoid the need to change their lifestyle. These patients have not yet accepted the fact that they will never be successful until they change their behavior. And the biggest behavior change is in eating. I'll talk about that next.

Eating Strategies

All human beings are sensory driven. We have five senses—taste, touch, smell, sight, and hearing—and to some extent we enjoy having each of them stimulated, sometimes all at the same time. When we go to the movies the experience includes not only the visual effects and the surround sound with volume up so that it literally moves us in our seats, but also the smell and taste of the popcorn. That's what I mean by stimulating all our senses at once.

Eating is one of the most enjoyable sensory-based activities in our lives. This is in no small part because it involves at least three of our five senses. Taste and smell are obvious, but don't discount the importance of the tactile sense, such as the smoothness of cream cheese, the crunch of a fresh taco, or the combination of textures in your favorite pizza. What's more, eating is something we can enjoy several times each day, and when we don't experience it we miss it. Is it any surprise that we have a tendency to overindulge, if for no other reason than to enjoy the experience?

Our enthusiasm for getting maximum sensory input is frequently manifested by eating as fast as possible. We take big bites of food, chew it a couple of times, and swallow. This is not because we are necessarily through with it as much as it is that we want the experience of the next bite. Each big bite is promptly followed by a similar big bite, often without a pause. We become automated eating machines, and what fuels the machine is the desire for sensory input.

Well, once the band is in place you will need to modify your love affair with the sensations of eating. This is not to say that you can't enjoy food, but the way you eat simply must change. What is interesting is that many patients say they actually enjoy food more when they slow down. While that may be true, I suspect for some the enjoyment comes from avoiding the discomfort that accompanies eating too fast.

The fact is that you, along with everyone else, enjoy putting food in your mouth. If you didn't, you wouldn't have a weight problem. This presents a major psychological problem once the band is in control of your portion size. Suddenly, instead of putting fork to mouth 30 or 40 times during a meal, and garnering all that sensory input, you are now down to what looks like no more than four or five bites. Even if your stomach is saying "I'm full," your sensory satisfaction center is crying out for more. The trick is to provide more sensory input without actually eating more. That is where smaller bites come in.

The tactic to keep yourself satisfied is to eat your small portion of food using the same number of bites you would normally have used to eat a large plate of food. Also, take at least the same amount of time to eat this small amount as you used to take to eat a large meal. Each time you put even a small amount of food in your mouth and chew it, be sure to experience the taste, the smell, and the texture.

Small bites also make it easier to chew the food into particles that are less likely to get stuck on the way down. Our dietitian tells patients to chew each bite until it is the consistency of apple sauce. Well, if you start out with a huge bite, by the time you chew it enough (if you can chew it enough) you are totally bored with it and it has lost all of its taste. Starting with small bites avoids this problem.

What Is a Small Bite?

If you're having trouble adjusting your bite size, get a baby spoon and put enough food on it to cover only the front half. Then chew this bite 15 to 20 times until it's the consistency of apple sauce before swallowing. Put your spoon or utensil down between bites. This is a great exercise to do every so often, especially if you find yourself having trouble with food coming back up.

What do we mean by small bites? Start with a baby spoon, and put enough food on it to cover only the front half. That sounds ridiculous I know, but it works. Remember, you are in training to develop new eating habits, so consider this a training exercise. Eventually, as you develop your new style of eating, you won't need the baby spoon. But I've had patients who occasionally need an eating refresher course with their trusty baby spoon.

Dr. Sewell's Golden Rules for AGB Patients*

- Eat until you are comfortable, NOT FULL!
- Choose protein first—you need 50 to 70 grams of protein per day.
- Eat slowly and chew your food well.
- Don't drink 15 minutes before or during meals, and avoid drinking for two hours after eating.
- Liquids will not satisfy your hunger, so you need to eat something.
- Exercise daily.

*This list is repeated from Chapter 9. Also, the 10 eating rules from a band manufacturer are listed on page 131.

All this sounds easy enough, right? Well, most of the time it is. But just like before surgery, there will be stress in your life and you'll feel the need for a release. There will be times when you feel depressed and you'll naturally seek comfort. Or when you achieve a goal, you'll still feel that you deserve a reward. In each of these situations, without even thinking, you will resort to what has always helped relieve your stress, raise your mood, or provide immediate gratification—food. But, with a band, if you resort to your usual eating habits, the results will be quite different than what you are used to. The band is going to let you know immediately if you eat too fast, eat too much, or don't chew your food adequately. It is your "drill sergeant" and is with you constantly.

When the small upper stomach pouch is full, you will sense you'd better not eat any more. The band is telling you that any additional food you swallow has no place to go. If you keep eating, the food will remain in the lower end of the esophagus. The muscles of the esophagus will continue to contract aggressively in an attempt to push everything through into the stomach. Since the band will not allow the food to pass through, this muscular effort creates tremendous pressure inside the esophagus. This leads first to a sense of fullness in your chest and throat and eventually causes chest pain. While that is going on, the lining of the esophagus is producing more mucus and the output of saliva is increased, both in an attempt to provide further lubrication to help the food pass.

There are only two ways to relieve the pressure from having food stuck in the lower esophagus: either wait until the food passes or bring it back up. When it comes up it isn't really like the kind of vomiting that you do with an upset stomach. It is less violent and generally more of a voluntary act. Patients describe it in a variety of terms, including spitting up, a productive burp, regurgitation, and others I've heard that I won't repeat. When the food comes up it is usually accompanied by considerable foaming mucus. Often the amount of food is relatively small, but the amount of mucus can be considerable. The message is clear—stop eating when you first get a sense of fullness.

While much of the time the problem of spitting up after eating is related to simply overeating, that is not always the case. I've had many patients tell me that they take only one or two bites before they experience the sensation of esophageal spasm and have to spit up what they just ate. Frequently that is followed by an ability to eat much better. This sounds strange, but it is such a common complaint that there must be a reason for it. While I have no proof, I suspect that what is happening is that the patient starts out with a couple of generous size bites, which quickly become stuck above the band. After they go through the uncomfortable process of spitting up these first couple of bites, they take much smaller bites, and thus avoid the previous result. Another possibility could be that their esophagus is initially highly sensitized to any food and spasms quickly with any resistance. The sensitivity may be diminished after the first material has been evacuated. Either way, this is a very common complaint among new band patients. It seems to improve over time, likely as a result of improved eating habits.

Many patients report a somewhat similar situation, stating that they are unable to tolerate anything to eat first thing in the morning. As a result they don't even attempt to eat until midmorning and sometimes not until early afternoon. The strange thing is that these same patients go on to relate that they can eat almost without restriction by their evening meal. Such a contrast must somehow be related to the effects of lying down through the night. Perhaps the esophagus fills up with mucus overnight and is incapable of fully emptying until the patient has been upright for several hours. The effects of gravity would aid in the passage of residual food and mucus out of the esophagus and into the stomach. This is purely speculation on my part, since I don't know the precise reason why so many patients report this phenomenon.

You Can Cheat the Band
G. Dick Miller, Psychologist

Patients are usually shocked when I tell them, "You can cheat the band." But you can, and people do it all the time. What I mean by cheating the band is that you can uncover ways to eat where there's little or no restriction. In other words, you can still find a way to abuse yourself with food and gain weight.

Why am I telling you this? Because you'll find out anyway. And because I want to acknowledge your right to choose. What the band gives you is the ability to make a decision about how you want your life to be. If you're looking for someone or something to "make" you behave the way you "should," with no regard for your choice in the matter, then you're setting yourself up for failure.

If this is scary for you, then you're still operating in your thinking under the old punishment paradigm—"threaten me, control me, tell me what I have to do." Under that paradigm we learn to dislike the task and the person who is requiring us to do the task. After we get done disliking all the people involved, we turn on ourselves, because that's the only person left. We rebel, and because we're in such a bad mood we're still hanging on the image of an adult that "should be able to do whatever they want to do." We haven't taken on the lifestyle change in a good spirit. We've been dragging ourselves, and that creates so much friction.

It doesn't have to be that way. But I see it all the time. People abuse themselves for failing, they go back and eat what they want to eat, they curse themselves, they abuse the diet, then they say it didn't work for them. In reality, they didn't have the kind of thinking that would work going in. They looked from the beginning for something outside themselves to "fix" them. Because, if you think about it, if you cheat the band, who are you really cheating?

What works is deciding to move from "have to" into "want to." From there it's only a short distance to the optimum thinking, which is "it's in my best interest to" or "it would be smart for me to."

What Best Describes Your Thinking?

- Do I have to?
- Do I want to?
- Is it in my best interest (or smart) to?

The truth is that you have options. Ask yourself, Am I willing to tell myself things that are not true, not consistent with my physical health and not consistent with my goals? Or am I willing to acknowledge that I have choices, take a look at them, and make a decision that's in my best interests? If you acknowledge your ability to opt for what you want, you don't have to feel resistance, resentment, or anger toward something or someone else. And then you're setting yourself up for success.

Choosing Foods for Success

To be successful with the AGB, patients need to train themselves to eat differently. The problem is that you have been used to eating way more than what is necessary. The total calorie intake of a morbidly obese person is almost always more than 3,000 calories per day. For some it may be as high as 5,000 calories per day or more. Because of their slow metabolic rate, most obese people don't even begin losing weight until their daily calorie intake falls below 2,000 calories per day, and for some that number is closer to 1,000 calories per day.

It isn't just a matter of calories. Your body needs certain nutrients every day, or nearly every day, in order to function properly. Starvation is not a good option. The dietitian can help you by providing a guide for what to eat and encourage new and better eating techniques, but the bottom line is that you still need to eat. The best approach is to have three small meals each day. It takes only a couple of ounces of food to fill the stomach pouch above the band. Any more and the problem of esophageal spasm and spitting up will occur. Since the volume is necessarily small, it is imperative to choose wisely what you eat to avoid malnutrition.

The most common form of malnutrition following any bariatric surgical procedure is protein deficiency. Your body needs protein, and if it doesn't get it from your diet it will take it from wherever it can get it, including your own muscles. We've all seen pictures of prisoners of war whose muscles have almost completely wasted away. If you look carefully at those pictures, you'll also notice that those emaciated prisoners have little or no hair. Protein is required to grow hair, and so one of the first signs of protein deficiency is hair loss, along with a thin and dull appearance to the remaining hair. That usually occurs long before significant muscle has been lost. Protein deficiency can be avoided by taking in 60 to 80 grams of protein each day. To help ensure adequate protein intake, we recommend that patients eat protein first at each meal.

Normal sources of protein include meat, eggs, fish, poultry, milk, cheese, beans, and nuts. For most Americans, red meat has been a primary source of protein all their lives. Certainly steaks and chops are great sources of protein, but they are also among the most difficult foods to chew into pieces small enough to pass through the band. So, instead of struggling with red meat, we encourage patients to eat protein-rich foods that are easier to chew, such as fish, chicken, and turkey. If their protein intake is still marginal, a protein bar is an excellent supplement. Some patients prefer protein shakes, but it is hard to get the same amount of protein from a shake as you get from a bar. An added benefit of the protein bar is that the solid material helps satisfy the need to chew something.

Recipes for Protein Shakes

(These recipes assume you have protein powder that provides 24 grams of protein per 1-ounce scoop.)

Note: Some people believe that adding a package of Splenda®, Sweet'n Low®, or other artificial sweetener to each recipe improves the flavor. Others find that to be too much sweetness. Much of this is personal preference, so try different amounts or other flavors of fat-free/sugar-free instant puddings.

Basic recipe:
In a blender:
Mix 8 oz. of water or more
6–8 ice cubes or more
2 scoops of protein shake powder
Then you may add the following:
1 strawberry, 2–3 raspberries, or 2–3 blueberries
1 tsp. vanilla extract
½ to 1 scoop of **sugar-free** gelatin, pudding, or Kool-Aid® (any flavor)
1 tsp. almond extract
1 tsp. instant coffee granules

¼ tsp. cinnamon
¼–½ tsp. lime or lemon juice
One-half can of diet soda
Nutrition information:
(300 calories, 48 grams of protein)

Vanilla/Cinnamon Shake

2 scoops vanilla protein powder
½ scoop fat-free/sugar-free (FF/SF)
    vanilla instant pudding mix (or to taste)
½ –1 tsp. vanilla extract
cinnamon to taste
Blend with water, then
Blend all with crushed ice
Nutrition information:
(300 calories, 48 grams of protein)

Pistachio Shake

2 scoops vanilla protein powder
½–1 scoop FF/SF pistachio instant pudding mix
½–1 tsp. almond extract
Blend with water, then
Blend all with crushed ice
Nutrition information:
(300 calories, 48 grams of protein)

Banana Shake

2 scoops vanilla protein powder
¾ scoop FF/SF banana instant pudding mix
½–1 tsp. vanilla extract
Blend with water, then
Blend all with crushed ice
Nutrition information:
(300 calories, 48 grams of protein)

Chocolate Shake

2 scoops chocolate protein powder
½ scoop FF/SF chocolate instant pudding mix
½–1 tsp. almond extract, if desired
Blend with water, then
Blend all with crushed ice
Nutrition information:
(300 calories, 48 grams of protein)

Protein Snack List

- One tablespoon peanut butter with two crackers.
- A quarter-cup 1 percent cottage cheese with a quarter-cup unsweetened fruit.
- One piece string cheese with a quarter-cup fresh fruit.
- One ounce reduced-fat cheese and two crackers.
- A half-cup sugar-free yogurt.
- One cup skim or 1 percent milk with one packet of Carnation instant breakfast (no sugar added).
- One hard boiled or scrambled egg with a few sprinkles of shredded cheese.
- One half of a small banana with one tablespoon of peanut butter.
- One tablespoon of peanut butter with one-half cup sugar-free instant pudding.
- A half-cup fat-free refried beans covered with a few sprinkles of reduced-fat shredded cheese.
- One half of an AdvanEdge® bar.
- Four to five medium-size steamed or boiled chilled shrimp with two tablespoons cocktail sauce.
- Lettuce wrap with 1 ounce lean, broiled, baked, or grilled chicken breast, turkey, or fish.
- One to two slices lean luncheon meat (chicken, turkey, ham) rolled up with a thin sliced pickle.
- Grilled tomato slices with two tablespoons shredded mozzarella or grated parmesan cheese.

Vitamins

Some people are convinced that by taking a handful of vitamins every day they will remain healthier. While that argument has been made by vitamin manufacturers for decades, I strongly discourage my patients from taking large doses of vitamins. Large vitamin pills can easily become lodged in the narrowed area of the stomach created by the band, obstructing it the same way a large bite of inadequately chewed food would.

Vitamin deficiencies can occur following AGB surgery, but these are far less likely than they are with other bariatric operations, such as gastric bypass. If you are eating anything close to a normal diet, it is unlikely that you will become deficient in any of the common vitamins. Nevertheless, we always recommend to our patients that they take a multivitamin supplement everyday. These come in chewable form, which reduces the possibility of the vitamin pill getting stuck in the band.

Taking in Fluids

For some patients the most challenging change to their typical eating behavior revolves around the need to avoid drinking liquids with their meals. Everybody is used to the idea of having a glass of water, tea, coffee, milk, juice, wine, or something liquid with their meal. However, to achieve success with the AGB, you need to drink fluid before your meal, and wait two hours after eating before drinking anything else. If every time you take a bite of food you "wash it down" with something to drink, you will liquefy the food you just ate. This will tend to "wash it through" the band, and you'll be able to eat much more than the small pouch should allow.

This new way of eating is more typical of animal behavior. Animals don't stop eating to go get a drink and then come back to their food. They drink when they are thirsty and they eat when they are hungry. Isn't it funny how you don't see many obese animals—unless, of course, they're under the direct care and feeding of a human being?

It is important to drink plenty of water; that means about 64 ounces a day. To accomplish this you'll need to drink a glass of water or tea before eating. If you wait until after you eat, the food in your pouch will not allow the liquids to pass through the area of the band. This is called the "cork effect." The result is similar to the productive burp, only it will be the water that comes up.

Kristen's Story

I discovered I had a thyroid problem as an adult. I was a normal size kid and teenager and never thought about having a weight problem. But I kept getting bigger and bigger, my bones were aching, and I was just busting at the seams. I got to 250 pounds, and I'm 5 feet, 3 inches with a BMI of 44.3.

I have a petite frame, and my knees, ankles, and feet were hurting so bad I could hardly walk. I kept justifying to myself that lots of people are bigger than me, but I couldn't ignore my huffing and puffing. So I started researching, found the band, and during the four years I tried to figure out how to get a band, I talked to everyone I could find about it.

Once I thought the band might work for me, at the beginning of my research, I talked to my dad about helping me pay for it. He said I must be crazy. I told him I was scared of diabetes or a stroke, and scared about the rest of my life being this way. His answer was for me to go on a diet and make it work. So I said okay. I tried diets and prescribed weight-loss drugs, but nothing worked.

Then I got married, and between the two of us, my husband and I, we found a way to pay for a band. So I went back to my dad and told him I was doing it no matter what. At that point, I found out that Dad was on the board of an insurance company and had heard a doctor talk about the band. So he said now he could talk to me about it. After we discussed it, he said he'd pay for part, so that's what we did.

I had my surgery on November 1 of 2005. That date is my wedding anniversary. I think it's great I got my band on such a very important date for me.

I did the pre-op diet. I called it the diet from hell. I did two weeks of no carbs, no vegetables that had sugar, and I was miserable. The day I went in to see the surgeon and start the pre-op diet, I told them I'd had a diet Dr. Pepper that morning, and they said that's the last one. So I got off carbonated drinks, too. I know people who have the band, and they told me carbonated drinks would stretch my new stomach. I wasn't willing to pay for the band and then sabotage myself. But that was one of the hardest things for me to give up.

There were no problems in the surgery. Afterward I did have the referred pain from the gas they used to inflate my abdomen, and the only way to get the gas out is walking. When I wasn't walking, I lay flat on my back and put a bunch of pillows under my legs. It was pretty painful for about two days. But even though I had the surgery on Thursday, I was back at work on Tuesday. Part of the reason I could do that is I have a sedentary job, and I don't have to do a lot of moving and lifting. The only thing I found myself doing was holding my port area at work before I even realized I was doing it, because I had some soreness there.

My first fill I was scared. I looked like a deer in the headlights. I told the nurse I was nervous and I don't like needles. I talked to other patients in the waiting room. I've decided it was the not knowing that terrified me. I waited five weeks before I had the first fill, even though my surgeon probably would have done it sooner because, from the beginning, I never felt like I had a band. Even after a couple of fills, I noticed I could still eat anything I wanted. It took several fills, every four weeks, over a few months' time, before I felt restriction. What I've found talking to people in my surgeon's waiting room while I'm sipping water after a fill is that fills are a very individual process. Everyone is different. I also found it's rare to find someone with no restriction post-op, like I had.

I have noticed that every time I get a fill, it's a learning process. I don't look at it as restriction because I don't like saying, "I can't eat this," and "I can't eat that." I prefer to concentrate on what works. I discovered that fresh ground turkey works well for me after this last fill. And I season it so it doesn't taste bland. Red meat doesn't work for me at all anymore. I enjoy looking for new menu items and recipes I can eat. I tell myself this is a learning process. If one thing doesn't work, I try something else. For example, if the chips and hot sauce don't work for me anymore at the Mexican place, I'll try chips and queso instead and stay focused on that. I want to move out of the place that got me here to begin with.

In the beginning, I did not exercise. I probably could have lost more by now, but I wasn't ready. I didn't want to exercise, but I took it on when I lost enough weight to start feeling better. I started walking and I joined the health club. My husband exercises with me. He's very supportive. We talk the whole time, and the exercise time passes quickly. I tell him, "You don't know what it's like to be fat and keep walking," and he encourages me. My endocrinologist likes it that I walk. He's watching my thyroid because of my weight loss, and he's adjusting my dosage levels downward.

I've always had lots and lots of friends, until I got so overweight, and then I went into hibernation. I was too embarrassed to see anyone. Now that my self-esteem is so much better, I promised my husband I'd get into my jeans and we'd start dancing. I think I'll come out as more of myself as I get more weight off. I've had issues with my mother, and my therapist told me as the weight comes off the issues will resurface.

I usually lose about 1 to 2 pounds a week. Sometimes I lose more. I just got under the 200 pound mark at my current weight of 198. I weigh only when I go to the surgeon's office, and that's on purpose. Weighing is a head game for me. When I dieted, I got to the point where I was obsessed with the scales, and I said to myself this is stupid. With the band, if I stay focused on doing what I'm supposed to do, I lose weight.

I love it that I got the band. It's given me a chance to bring myself back. I was hopeless at the time I had it done. Some people who've been overweight most of their life look at their weight differently than someone like me, who became overweight as an adult. I'd say to myself, Why can't I go to the beach and have fat on me and be perfectly happy like that lady over there who is having a great time? But I couldn't. So now I feel like I got myself back.

Conclusion

Learning to eat with an AGB and avoid the problems discussed here is not easy. Many patients struggle for months before they begin to understand that it isn't really about the band, it's about them. It's about changing behavior. Changing any habit, especially something as firmly ingrained as the way we eat, is a truly daunting challenge. The band is there to help guide you through this change, but it won't make the change for you. You must do the changing yourself. When you do, the rewards can be incredible. As we'll discuss in the next chapter, improved health, better mobility, and a richer, fuller, life unencumbered by obesity make all the hard work worthwhile. But, just as important, is the personal satisfaction of knowing you are the instrument of your own success.

11

The Health Benefits of the AGB and Weight Loss

Formulate and stamp indelibly on your mind a mental picture of yourself as succeeding. Hold this picture tenaciously. Never permit it to fade. Your mind will seek to develop the picture. . . . Do not build up obstacles in your imagination.

—Dr. Norman Vincent Peale

In the last chapter, we looked at adjustments and the eating strategies that will make you successful with the band. In this chapter, we look at the payoff for that success. What can you realistically expect in terms of improvement to your health? It is true that some band patients experience the disappearance of high blood pressure, sleep apnea, and other debilitating illnesses. They can potentially experience the permanent remission of other illnesses such as diabetes. But just how is that possible? And how do health improvements with the AGB compare with those of other weight-loss surgical options? Let's take a look.

Factors That Influence the Improvement of Your Health

Patients seek out bariatric surgery for a variety of reasons, but in my experience it is health concerns that provide the compelling reason why obese individuals may be wise to consider weight-loss surgery. The objective should be improved health, not weight loss just for the sake of weight loss. At the same time, most patients are justifiably concerned about the health risks that naturally accompany procedures such as the gastric bypass. This is why many choose the AGB as a lower-risk alternative. But the question that must be asked is, What about the results?

Improved health following any bariatric operation depends on a number of factors. One of the most obvious is the amount of weight lost. The rapidity of the weight loss also can play a role, and faster is not necessarily better. There is no question that weight loss following gastric bypass is typically faster and more dramatic than it is after the AGB. Those patients who undergo gastric bypass may have a quicker improvement in some of their health problems than patients undergoing AGB, but at the same time they are somewhat more likely to have other problems related to malnutrition.

Following a gastric bypass, patients may lose as much as 5 pounds per week or more. They tend to lose the majority of their weight during the first six months and then begin to taper off. During this time it is very important to follow a diet with plenty of protein to avoid hair loss and maintain muscle mass. They must also take vitamin B12 regularly to avoid anemia, since iron cannot be utilized by the body to make red blood cells without vitamin B12.

AGB patients tend to lose the majority of their weight over a year or two at a slower and steadier rate, usually about a pound to a pound and a half per week. They too need to be on a high-protein diet, but they typically have less trouble maintaining adequate nutrition. Since the stomach is not bypassed, they don't require B12 supplements. When we look at the results over three to five years, the two procedures actually offer quite similar weight-loss outcomes.

With weight loss, both gastric bypass and AGB patients can experience significant improvement in a variety of medical ailments including diabetes, high blood pressure, sleep apnea, reflux, and various back and joint pains. However, weight loss is not a cure-all! Some patients continue to suffer from one or more of these conditions despite losing significant amounts of weight. In other words, there is more to being healthy than just controlling your weight. But, more often than not, for morbidly obese people virtually all health problems become easier to manage once they have lost weight.

Improvement in Diabetes

Diabetes is a complex metabolic illness, characterized by problems processing the simple sugar glucose. Many people still refer to it as "sugar diabetes." The actual medical term is diabetes mellitus, which differentiates this disease from another illness, diabetes insipidus, a disorder involving excess water loss through the kidneys. In general, when people, including physicians, use the term "diabetes," they are referring to diabetes mellitus.

To further complicate matters there are two forms of diabetes mellitus, Type 1 and Type 2. In both types the fundamental problem involves levels of glucose in the bloodstream that are significantly higher than they should be.

Type 1 diabetes has historically been called juvenile onset diabetes, or hereditary diabetes, because it commonly occurs in younger patients and tends to run in families. In recent years the name has been changed to Type 1 diabetes, because not all patients are young, nor do they have a family history of the disease. This form of diabetes is influenced to some extent by obesity, and obese patients with Type 1 disease are encouraged to lose weight. But most people with Type 1 diabetes are not morbidly obese. Type 1 patients virtually all require insulin, either by injection or by intravenous pump.

Type 2 diabetes is the more common variety (90–95 percent), and is the one most closely associated with obesity. This form of diabetes, Type 2, will be the subject of the remainder of this discussion.

Glucose is the number one source of energy for the cells of our body, but for the cells to use glucose the sugar molecule must first be absorbed into the cell. Insulin, a chemical produced by specialized cells in the pancreas, facilitates that process.

Patients who have diabetes don't process glucose normally. A simple way to understand diabetes is to think of it as either not enough insulin, or to think that the insulin present is simply not effective because the cells have become resistant to its effects. In either case, more glucose remains in the bloodstream because less is taken up by the cells. Obviously, this process is much more complicated, but for purposes of our discussion, it will do.

The association between obesity and diabetes is well known, but the precise mechanism by which obesity seems to "cause" diabetes is not completely understood. What we do know in general is that fatty tissue tends to be more resistant to insulin than other tissue types, so the transport of glucose into fat cells is impaired. With increasing weight gain this difference becomes exaggerated, and the patient's blood sugar increases. If you are diagnosed with diabetes or even pre-diabetes, one of the first things your doctor will tell you is that you need to lose weight. So once again we get back to the issue of voluntary weight loss. Pre-diabetes is simply defined as having higher than normal blood glucose levels, but not high enough to meet the criteria required for the condition to be called diabetes.

The diagnosis of Type 2 diabetes signals the start of a race to control this serious disease before it has time to cause any of the well-recognized pathologic effects. These include diabetic retinopathy, the leading cause of blindness, and diabetic nephropathy, the leading cause of kidney failure. Also high on the list of problems associated with diabetes are coronary artery disease and cerebral vascular disease, with heart attack and stroke being the leading causes of death among patients with diabetes. The effects of peripheral vascular disease, including potential limb loss, are known to be greatly accelerated by diabetes. Diabetes also interferes with nerve function, causing what is called diabetic neuropathy. This is the underlying cause of disabling diabetic foot ulcers. It is also well recognized that people with diabetes don't fight infection well, and typically they don't heal injuries or surgical wounds as well as those without diabetes. The bottom line is this: you need to get your diabetes under control, because there are a lot of bad things that are likely to happen if you don't.

Obviously, diabetes is a huge problem and has been on the rise in the United States for several decades. Not surprisingly, this increase parallels the rise in obesity in our society. According to governmental statistics from 2005, nearly 21 million Americans have diabetes, with nearly one-third of those currently undiagnosed. Perhaps even more alarming is the fact that nearly 10 percent of Americans over the age of 20 now have diabetes, with the highest prevalence being among American Indians and Alaskan Natives at about 18 percent each, as well as the Hispanic and black populations at about 14 percent. In 2002, the medical cost associated with treating diabetes in the United States was estimated at $92 million, making it one of the most costly of all diseases.

While these statistics are frightening, the good news is that most obese patients who are able to lose weight successfully will experience a significant improvement in their diabetes. But, as you know, losing weight can be an extremely difficult task. Many patients who have diabetes require medication to lower their blood sugar, and an unfortunate side effect of artificially lowering blood sugar is often an increased appetite. This creates a vicious circle in which obesity leads to the need for medication, and medications lower blood sugar, which in turn increases appetite. Increased appetite results in excessive eating, driving glucose levels higher and causing weight gain, leading to the need for even more medication. Eventually the diabetes can become impossible to control with diet and oral medications alone, so patients end up being placed on insulin.

One of the major objectives of any bariatric operation in a patient with diabetes is to break the cycle of excess weight, medication, hunger, and further weight gain. In some cases following weight-loss surgery patients are able to eliminate their medications, and diabetes often ceases to be a problem. This is particularly true for patients who have had diabetes for less than five years, and for those who are not taking insulin. For those who have had diabetes for many years, especially if they have been on insulin injections for several years, it is less likely that they will ever be completely cured of their diabetes. But, even under these circumstances it is quite common for patients to experience a significant reduction in their insulin dosage.

A variety of reports in the medical literature have documented diabetes improvement following gastric bypass surgery, with some demonstrating total resolution in 75 percent of patients and either resolution or significant improvement in more than 90 percent. The results reported following the AGB are not quite as spectacular. They are more in the 50 to 60 percent range for total resolution, and 80 to 90 percent resolution or significant improvement in diabetes. Sometimes the facts are difficult to separate from the hype that can accompany what should be a nonbiased scientific study. Regardless, there is clear and unquestioned evidence that shows that when patients lose weight they more often than not experience a significant improvement in their diabetes.

What is interesting is how fast this improvement in diabetes can occur following surgical procedures that restrict your ability to eat, such as the AGB. Improvement is generally seen long before major weight loss has occurred. For many years diabetes educators have preached to their patients to follow a diet of fewer than 1,800 calories to lower blood sugar. Following the AGB procedure, that is precisely what happens. Patients simply can't eat they way they used to, making it difficult to take in as many calories, so their blood sugar goes down.

Immediately after surgery I place all my patients with diabetes on a low-calorie liquid diet, and we monitor their blood glucose level every six hours. Typically the levels are much lower than the patient had expected. They almost always express concern over the fact that they haven't taken their diabetes medication, even though I've explained that it is all right to be off their medication. They won't need to take medication unless or until their blood sugar starts to go back up. I have them monitor their sugars closely once they go home, and most are surprised at how well controlled they continue to be on the postoperative diet. Obviously, that is not the case with every patient, especially those who are on insulin, but even patients on insulin will almost always have to adjust their dosage down.

Longer-term the results following AGB in patients with diabetes are extremely promising, but they depend on a continuing commitment to a change in lifestyle. In addition to weight loss, getting exercise and following a sensible diet are vital components of diabetes management.

Whitney's Story

I was diagnosed with Type 2 diabetes a year before I got the band. I was 326 pounds and I'm 5 feet, 10 inches. Every woman in my family had diabetes, so I got really scared. I'm a full-time nurse and I've seen a lot of what diabetes can do to someone, so I decided that my eyes, my feet, and my kidneys were not worth that extra Twinkie®.

It was my endocrinologist who found the diabetes. I gained 50 pounds in a year and was concerned about how I had gained so quickly. I was planning my wedding, was a full-time nurse, and was going to graduate school, so it wasn't like I was idle. The weight wouldn't come off no matter what I did, and the endocrinologist said I needed to do something quickly to lose the weight. I found Dr. Sewell, went to one of his seminars, talked to him, and got to know his staff. I battled insurance companies a lot. Even though mine said the band was a covered benefit, they refused to pay for it. I had 300 pages of documentation on failed weight-loss attempts, knee surgery, and the diabetes. I finally decided that my health was too important to continue to wait, so I decided to pay for my own band.

I'm a labor and delivery nurse, and I've seen some train wrecks with pregnant bypass patients. I was terrified of that for myself. I thought the adjustability of the band was a cool option as well.

I was on the pre-op diet for the last two weeks of my school semester. I really committed to the diet, and as a result, my need for the diabetes medication diminished. The endocrinologist took me off the medication, and I have never needed it again.

I was banded in August of 2003, and in a year I'd lost 94 pounds. By then I was married and found out I was pregnant. Dr. Sewell is very conservative when it comes to the management of pregnant women, and he took all the fluid out of my band. I had a high-risk pregnancy with lots of complications. My daughter was born premature, but she's happy and healthy. A week after I delivered in March of 2005, he put 1.0cc back in, but he didn't reinflate the band back to my previous level until I was done breast feeding.

While I'm so happy with my healthy baby, I haven't gotten back to where I was before the fill was taken out. Right now I'm down 65 pounds from my pre-op weight. I still yo-yo. I find having a band is a lot of headwork. I had never been thin my whole life, so when people started paying attention to me, I thought, "Was I that much of a mutant before?" It's great to be appreciated, but it's also nice to know there are other things people value you for.

I hate exercise. I don't do it. And I have bad knees and suffered a bad ankle sprain this year. Plus I'm so tired. My baby is now 19 months, and I think that's part of it.

It's weird being a band patient and having a kid. I think I may overcompensate, like making sure we don't celebrate with food, that we don't comfort ourselves with food when we're sad and all that. Looking at my family history, everything good happened around a big table of food. My dad is from a big Southern family, and everything was made from scratch, never processed or out of a box.

Currently, I'm struggling with my band. There is stress in my GI system, and Dr. Sewell and I are trying to rule out GERD. I am frustrated. I want the control the band gave me back again. I had an upper GI and still we can't figure out what's wrong. Dr. Sewell doesn't know exactly what the deal is. I'm his challenge. Even so, I don't regret getting the band, but I think I'd change the way I managed my pregnancy. Instead of taking all the fill out, I'd have just some taken out. I equate my problems with when it was deflated during my pregnancy.

I've really tried to stay focused spiritually and believe that the problems I'm having now are something God is putting me through to teach me something. I work with a lot of people, and I often ended up telling them about the band usually just through casual conversation. I give them good and reliable information, and that's pretty powerful. I can't tell you how many people have come back to me to let me know they or a family member got a band. But I tell them about my struggles, too.

Has my band journey been easy for me? No. Do I wish I'd had a totally uneventful, uncomplicated course? Yes. But I'd do it again.

Improvement in Hypertension
(The Silent Killer)

"Hypertension" is the medical term for what most people call high blood pressure. To grasp the importance of this common condition requires a basic understanding of the cardiovascular system, starting with your heart. The heart is the engine that drives the body. It pumps blood through the lungs where red blood cells pick up oxygen. It then pumps this oxygen-loaded blood out to all areas of the body through a system of vessels, called arteries. As oxygen is delivered to all the tissues, carbon dioxide is picked up and carried back to the heart through a vast network of veins. The blood is immediately sent back through the lungs, where the carbon dioxide is exchanged for oxygen, completing the circuit.

Your heart beats on average about 70 times per minute over your entire life, maintaining the constant flow of oxygen and nutrients to every part of your body. This system requires no thought on your part and continues uninterrupted for 80, 90, or even 100 years or more, making it one of the most amazing aspects of life.

Obviously, there are a number of things that can influence how well this system works, and one of the most important factors is the pressure of the blood

within the arteries. If your blood pressure is too low, blood may not get to certain areas, such as the brain. A transient episode of low blood pressure can
cause you to faint. If the blood pressure remains low for a prolonged period, it
causes shock and even death if vital organs don't get enough oxygen. By contrast, if your blood pressure is too high it may cause few if any immediate symptoms. Sometimes patients will report a headache or a pounding sensation, but
most of the time high blood pressure is a silent problem, and over time it can be
a silent killer.

Blood pressure is measured in millimeters of mercury and is generally
recorded as two numbers, such as 120 over 80. The first number is called the
systolic pressure, the peak pressure that exists when the heart is actively contracting to push blood through the arteries. The second number is called the diastolic pressure, the minimum pressure that remains within the arteries during
that period between heartbeats.

The heart works best when the blood pressure is maintained within the normal range. When the pressure is higher than normal, the heart is required to
push against considerably more resistance. Over time this can create pump
problems as the heart muscle enlarges to compensate. An enlarged heart is less
efficient and can eventually lead to heart failure.

Hypertension also causes damage to the arteries themselves. The wall of the
arteries will compensate to this increased pressure by a thickening of the wall
and narrowing of the channel, a process known as arteriosclerosis, or peripheral
vascular disease. It used to be called "hardening of the arteries," which is actually a pretty good description of what these vessels become—hard. Each and
every artery in the body can be affected, but some are more susceptible than
others, including the arteries to the heart (coronary artery disease) and the
brain (cerebral vascular disease). When enough narrowing occurs in these arteries, it can lead to heart attack and stroke.

Other factors certainly play a role in the development of arteriosclerosis, including diabetes, and when combined with hypertension the result is pre-
dictably bad. One of the most frightening statistics is that nearly three out of
four adults with diabetes also have high blood pressure.

The bottom line is that high blood pressure is a silent killer. But it doesn't
have to be. Most of the time hypertension can be controlled through weight
loss, reducing salt intake, and increasing physical exercise. (Sound familiar?)
When those efforts are not successful, it becomes necessary to add one or more
medications to lower the blood pressure artificially.

Obesity is a well-recognized and often major factor in the development of
hypertension. Volumes have been written about this association, but there is no
consensus on exactly how the two are related. Many researchers believe that el-

evated blood pressure in obese patients is related to the kidneys retaining too much sodium. In simple terms this means that obese people tend to retain salt and retain water, which leads to an increased blood pressure. Certainly it is far more complicated than that, but there appears to be a direct correlation between obesity and hypertension in many patients.

It naturally follows then that losing weight should result in lowering of the blood pressure, and that is what we generally see. As is the case with diabetes, there are many articles in the medical literature documenting this fact. Losing weight with the AGB results in resolution of hypertension in about half of patients, meaning that they are able to get off medication entirely. Nearly three out of four are either resolved or are more easily controlled once they have lost weight.

Like the improvement in diabetes, the reduction in blood pressure often doesn't take very long. The restricted diet after surgery also tends to restrict both salt and water intake, so we watch the blood pressure closely in the hospital after surgery, then have the patient monitor it closely at home.

I distinctly recall one patient who returned to see me in the office one week after undergoing an AGB procedure. When he came in he looked terrible. He was unsteady on his feet and could barely stand. We took him into the exam room and checked his blood pressure. It was 80 over 40! That's low! Obviously my first thoughts included some delayed operative complication such as bleeding or infection. His abdomen was soft, and he denied having any pain. When I asked him if he was taking his blood pressure medication, he informed me, "Oh yes! My doctor told me years ago that I would have to take that for the rest of my life." I explained to him that it was the medication that was causing the problem, and that he should stop taking it. I wanted to admit him to the hospital, but he was insistent on going home. I convinced him to come back two days later, which he did, and by that time his blood pressure was normal at 120 over 80 and he felt fine.

This all sounds too good to be true, right? A surgical procedure that "cures" high blood pressure? Well, the fact is that even if your blood pressure falls to normal after AGB surgery, hypertension can return unless—are you ready for this?—you get regular exercise and eat a sensible diet. This is not rocket science!

Improvement in Sleep Apnea (The Thief in the Night)

Many obese patients report that they are tired all the time. It is easy to pass off this chronic fatigue as the direct result of carrying around all those extra pounds, and that certainly plays a part. But obesity can frequently lead to fatigue by interfering with sleep. A condition known as sleep apnea is quite common among obese patients, and it is often the "thief in the night" that robs you of a good night's sleep.

There are several stages of sleep, but the one that offers the most rest is called REM sleep, or Rapid Eye Movement sleep. During this deepest phase of sleep the body relaxes completely, and during this time we not only regenerate our body physically but we also recharge our psyche—we dream. Many morbidly obese individuals never reach this phase of sleep because as they begin to relax their airway becomes obstructed and they literally stop breathing, which causes them to wake up. Typically patients are not even aware of these episodes, because they immediately fall back to sleep. This can happen over and over, all night long. In the morning they "wake-up" still exhausted and remain tired throughout the day. They may be so tired that they even fall asleep at times during the day.

The medical term for this situation is Pickwickian syndrome, named for the character Joe in Charles Dickens's first popular novel, *The Pickwick Papers*. Joe was a very obese young man who was described as eating large quantities of food, then suddenly falling asleep anywhere, anytime. Patients who are so extremely obese that they can't walk or even get out of bed are at risk of dying from what amounts to a respiratory arrest as carbon dioxide builds up in their blood.

Snoring is closely related to sleep apnea and is also very common among obese patients; just ask their spouses! As you fall asleep and begin to relax the tissues in the throat and nasal passages tend to collapse in on your airway. The rhythmic movement of air through these partially blocked passages can create enough noise to keep the entire household awake!

Many remedies have been used to treat sleep apnea and snoring, including even surgical removal of the loose tissues in the back of the throat. But for those with proven sleep apnea, the most effective treatment is often a breathing assist device called a CPAP machine (Continuous Positive Airway Pressure) or a BiPAP machine (Bilevel Positive Airway Pressure). The patient wears a tight-fitting mask over the face that provides a small amount of positive pressure inside the upper airway. This pressure holds the passages open, allowing air to move in and out more easily.

Once you get used to wearing the mask these devices can provide major relief from the problem of sleep apnea and snoring. The results are often so dramatic that patients tell me they will not travel anywhere without their machine. One patient said that he will not go camping with his family unless they go somewhere with electricity for his CPAP machine. Obviously there is nothing like a good night's sleep.

While these machines can provide obese patients relief from sleep apnea, it is also possible to get dramatic results following weight-loss surgery. Typically, improvement comes after losing only 20 or 30 pounds. Patients tell me that they are not only sleeping better but also dreaming again, many for the first time in years. However, the most common statement I hear after weight-loss surgery is "I have so much more energy!"

Undoubtedly, some of this renewed energy is a direct result of not having to carry around so much excess weight, but most patients experience this phenomenon long before it should be expected based on their lighter load alone. Because they are finally getting some rest at night, they are waking up more refreshed and able to function through the day without that sense of chronic fatigue.

In a 2001 study of morbidly obese patients by Dr. Dixon and his colleagues from Australia, 59 percent of men and 45 percent of women suffered from various sleep disturbances prior to having AGB surgery. The group lost an average of 48 percent of their excess body weight during the first year after surgery. Snoring had been a major problem for 82 percent of these patients before surgery, but 12 months later only 14 percent reported that they still had a snoring problem. The incidence of sleep apnea decreased from 33 percent to only 2 percent. Daytime sleepiness fell from 39 percent to 4 percent, and only 2 percent of patients reported poor sleep quality, compared with 39 percent before the surgery. It would be interesting to see the results of a study of the sleeping patterns of their spouses, whose nights are no longer spent nudging their partner and urging them to "roll-over!"

Improvement in the Painful Load

For most people it is hard even to imagine lifting 100 pounds, yet morbidly obese people do that, and often more, without even thinking about it. They have adapted to carrying around far more weight than would seem possible, in large part because the weight has been added over a period of time. Their muscles have gradually enlarged to lift the load, but what about the bones and joints of their skeleton?

Our skeleton is designed to support our own normal weight, with built-in capacity that allows us to lift and strain against considerably more weight over short periods. The problem with obesity is that we can't put that extra weight aside and let our body rest. The bones and joints are subjected to near maximum stress continuously. Over time the wear and tear on the back, hips, knees, ankles, and feet are predictable.

Back Pain

The spine is the central support for the entire skeleton, and it also provides protection for the spinal cord. The nerves that go to every part of the body exit the column of bones, called vertebrae, through small openings, called foremen. The vertebra are stacked one on top of the other, extending from the end of the torso to the base of the skull. There are 8 cervical (neck), 12 thoracic (chest), 5 lumbar (lower back), and 5 sacral (pelvic) vertebrae. With the exception of the sacral vertebra, which are fused into one solid plate of bone forming the back of the pelvis, each vertebra is separated from the one above and the one below by a firm but spongy cushion called an intervertebral disc.

The bony parts of the spine can withstand tremendous pressure without breaking, in part because the discs compress like a shock absorber. When subjected to extreme pressure, however, a disc can rupture, putting pressure directly on the spinal cord or on one of the nerves. Depending on which disc it is and the severity of the disruption, the result can be neck pain, back pain, leg pain, or even numbness or weakness in one arm or leg. Morbid obesity increases the risk of this type of spine injury because excess weight creates excess pressure on each disc.

Chronic back pain is quite common among obese patients, but most of them don't have ruptured discs. Their pain is due to the constant strain on the muscles and tendons that support the spine.

Most obese patients with chronic back pain report improvement after losing only 15 to 20 pounds. If the pain is due to a ruptured disc or arthritis in the spine, losing weight may or may not lead to any improvement. These problems may require additional treatment, including even surgery. But if you ask any back surgeon, they will tell you that the results following a spinal operation of any kind are better after the patient has lost weight.

Foot, Ankle, Knee, and Hip Pain

Perhaps no other part of the body takes more punishment than your feet. They must bear every ounce of your weight as they literally "pound the pavement." Ankle joints are likewise subjected to compression with each step. The knee joints are extremely active, and the surfaces of the bones are protected by only thin wedges of cartilage. The hip joint is also subjected to tremendous stress. Given the mechanics of walking, is it any wonder that these areas of the body are the sites of frequent aches and pains? Add 100 pounds or more to the equation and you have a recipe for major problems.

Researchers have shown that during walking, each pound you weigh results in 4 pounds of pressure on your knee joints. That may not sound like much until you do the math. If you are 100 pounds overweight and take only 3,000 steps per day (less than 2 miles), the total pressure on your knees is a whopping 1.2 million pounds. That's per day! The result of this crushing load can accelerate arthritis, cartilage deterioration, and disabling pain. In other words, being obese wears out your joints far faster than normal. In sporting terms, it puts you on the sidelines.

Our bodies were designed to be mobile, and one of the most devastating effects of morbid obesity is immobility. I have had several patients who were using a cane, a walker, a wheelchair, or a scooter to help them get into my office for their initial evaluation. The irony is that everyone tells you to exercise to lose weight. Once you reach a certain point, however, and it is different for everyone, you are unable to exercise. It is simply too painful.

One solution is to have that painful hip or knee replaced. When you go to the orthopedic surgeon, the first thing you are told is, "You need to lose some weight before we can do your surgery." Doesn't anybody understand? The fact is that having a knee or hip replacement without losing weight makes it unlikely for the surgery to be successful. In fact, many of my patients are actually referred to me by their orthopedic surgeon for AGB surgery to improve the likelihood of a successful joint replacement. Occasionally, patients are able to delay or even avoid these operations by losing most of the weight that caused the joint pain to begin with. For those who go on to joint replacement, the speed and ease of their recovery, as well as their ultimate rehabilitation, are directly proportional to the amount of weight they have lost.

One of the most emotional events that I have had the privilege of witnessing in the past several years involved a morbidly obese woman who had been confined to a wheelchair for more than two years because of severe hip pain. She surprised us all about three months after her AGB surgery when she walked, with a cane, into the office. She had lost less than 30 pounds, but that was enough to allow her to regain an element of personal mobility.

Jack's Story

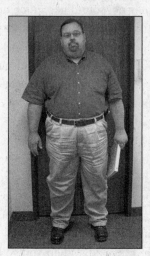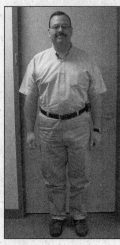

(Left) Jack, pre-op, 430 pounds.

(Right) Jack, 10 months post-op, 220 pounds.

I guess we all have that epiphany moment or that thing that pushes us over the edge. I was 6 feet, 2 inches and weighed 430 pounds. Once every month or two when I'd fly, there would be a stewardess or a flight attendant who would dig a seat belt extender out of the cabinet and give it to me. But once when I was trying to wedge myself into the seat, the attendant said, "Next time you may have to buy two tickets."

I had a lot of problems. I was having trouble with my knees and had a handicapped tag for my car. My doctor told me that if I didn't do something about my weight I'd be diabetic. I had sleep apnea, my blood pressure was poor, and my cholesterol was terrible. But nothing motivated me like what the flight attendant said. That was one of those little things that went all over me.

The next day I started my "quest," as you might call it. I looked into several options for a surgical solution, including the band and gastric bypass. I decided to go the band route, found Dr. Sewell, and went to one of his seminars. The night of the seminar I made an appointment, and two weeks later I started the whole process.

When Dr. Sewell put me on the pre-op diet we'd hoped for 8 to 10 pounds weight loss, and I lost 16. My surgery was in May of 2005, and that went well, too. I remember waking up in recovery and there was a little more pain than I'd anticipated, but I'd never had abdominal surgery before. I had the surgery on a Thursday and went back to work at the forensic laboratory on Monday.

I've had a lot of lifestyle changes, most of which were self-choices, such as that I decided not to do red meat at all. It's not a have-to thing, just a healthy choice I made. I stay away from pasta and potatoes. I drank a lot of carbonated stuff before, and that was a tough change for me. So now, if I want a Diet Coke® I open it up, let it go flat, and drink it the next day. The no drinking thing at a meal was a real big change for me, too. There were a lot of minor changes, but once I made up my mind to do it, then I just did it. I consider it a very minor trade-off for the benefits.

Right now, 16 months out, I've lost 210 pounds. I was in a size 52, and now I'm in a 38 pant. Every time I have to change my size down, I wait until the very last possible moment, because clothes are expensive.

My regular doctor is pretty amazed at where I am now health-wise. He was skeptical and not very supportive when I told him what I wanted to do. He's been very supportive now, though. The need for all the medications I was taking is gone, and he's definitely a believer. He says I should be the poster child for the band.

In the first six to eight months I didn't change my physical activity level a lot. After the pounds came off, I'm a lot more active now than I ever was. I started biking and I play soccer. I've added activity a little bit here and there. I have to pay to park and I now am in a lot farther away, where I save myself 40 bucks a month. I always park at the back of the parking lot now and walk, when before I parked in the handicapped spot.

I've revised my weight-loss goals downward three times. And I think I'll do it again and lose another 10 pounds to give myself a cushion. I'm still amazed every time I look in the mirror. And I'm still thankful. I experience good physical health, and I feel better about myself than I have in years. Everyone notices a change. The band has been a perfect choice for me.

Improvement in Gastroesophageal Reflux Disease (GERD)

If you watch television for more than a few minutes, you are bound to see an advertisement for one of a number of medications purporting to eliminate heartburn. That is because heartburn is extremely common, and the sale of these drugs is in the billions of dollars each year. Heartburn, also known as acid reflux, is caused by stomach acid backing up into the esophagus. More often than not this is due to failure of a valve at the lower end of the esophagus that should prevent stomach contents from going up the esophagus.

In some patients, simple heartburn progresses to what is called gastroesophageal reflux disease, or GERD. The chronic reflux of stomach contents up into your esophagus and the back of your throat can lead to a variety of other symptoms, including regurgitation of food, chest pain, asthma, laryngitis, bronchitis, pneumonia, sinus infections, and even dental problems. It can also damage the esophagus by forming ulcers, strictures, and even a premalignant condition known as Barrett's esophagus.

When properly placed, the AGB is actually quite effective in the management of GERD. It acts as another barrier to the movement of stomach contents up into the esophagus. Most patients are able to stop taking their heartburn medications immediately following surgery, but that is not always the case. In fact, if the band is placed too low, or if it slips down on the stomach, it can actually make symptoms of reflux worse. This is one of the complications of the AGB and will be covered in more detail in the next chapter.

Like all the medical problems discussed here, obesity is a major contributing factor in the development of GERD. In this instance it's because of the extra pressure on the abdomen, which can literally push stomach contents up into the esophagus. So, when treating patients for GERD, the first thing the gastroenterologist is going to say is, "Lose weight."

Am I a Fraud?
G. Dick Miller, Psychologist

When I work with band patients, I find they often feel like frauds. But it takes some time to get them to be honest enough to reveal this. Let me tell you how I usually get this information.

One of the questions each new group asks is, "How much do I tell about having a band?" People want to know if they should tell their coworkers, their family, their friends. And I ask, "Why are you not telling?"

Various answers come up. One is that I don't want pressure to perform, and if people know I have a band they'll have expectations. Another is that it's no one's business. Yet another is that I don't want to fail.

As we discuss this, it always comes up that members of the group view not telling as dishonest. But it depends on who you're not telling and why. If you opt not to tell people you work with, that's not any more dishonest than if you had hemorrhoid surgery and you didn't tell, or gas last night and you kept it to yourself. It's not dishonest to accept a compliment and not spill your entire life story.

But what I hear when people get really honest is that they feel like a phony if they don't tell. When they're losing weight and changing, they start hearing things like, "You look marvelous," and how well they are doing. And they think it's a cheat, like they're tricking people. In other words, they feel like a fraud.

Most of them felt that way going in. They decided from the beginning that the band is a fraud, a cheat, a way to do weight loss without doing the work. But they decided they'll trade the money for the band rather than being fat. Since they've paid so much money for it, they expect the band to do all the work. The surprise comes when they find out there's work on their end. And when they find out that they have to do work, too, then they feel cheated. One thing I hear a lot is, "I paid all this money, this thing should just work and I shouldn't have to do anything."

As I've said before, the band is simply a library card. All it does is get you into the place where you can do the necessary and required change. But when the patient changes, because they thought it was a fraud going in, often they won't give themselves credit. They say things like, "It was too easy," or they discount their own part in this for some other reason.

But it's not a fraud. You and your doctor made a decision for your health. Look at it this way. If a heart patient has bypass surgery and starts thinking better, working out, and changes their eating habits, they accept the compliment when someone tells them they look great. They don't feel guilty, like a fraud, like they tricked someone. But because we're talking weight loss and you got help, that doesn't mean you're a fraud any more than the heart patient.

What I see is a lot of shame, because we have a history. People say to themselves, "I've attempted many things to control myself in regard to food and weight. I've cheated with my food and now I've cheated with the band. So I am not going to give or allow myself full credit for making a rational decision about the band."

That's rotten self-talk, and it won't work for you. Give yourself credit, tell the people you feel comfortable with telling and graciously accept the compliments. This isn't a trick and it isn't a cheat. You can allow yourself full credit because you searched until you found a tool that worked for your weight loss, you did the inside work on yourself to make use of the tool, and now you're enjoying the results. Let that in.

Obesity Is Misunderstood

The pattern here should be obvious by now. No matter which physician you see, primary care or specialist, from cardiologist to spine surgeon, from pulmonologist to endocrinologist, invariably the first thing you're told is, "You need to lose weight." Unfortunately, they don't usually tell you how you are supposed to do that.

This may sound a bit harsh, but most physicians simply say, "Diet and get more exercise." Don't they realize that number one, you know that, and number two, you've tried that? Why is it that most physicians are so hesitant to recommend bariatric surgery, despite the fact that it is the only treatment with proven long-term results? I think in large part it is because the problem of obesity remains so misunderstood, plus the "cause" is easily passed back to the patient. It's your fault. It's a behavioral issue. It's a social issue. It's not a disease. It also seems that whenever the subject of weight-loss surgery is brought up in medical circles, the discussion is usually more about the risks of surgery than it is about the benefits.

The explosion of interest in bariatric surgery over the last decade is in no small part the result of patients taking a more active role in their own health. I have had patients come to my office with reams of printed information off the Internet. Some of it is applicable to their situation and some isn't, but the fact is that they are attempting to make an informed decision about health issues they recognize as important. This is a far cry from the days of my youth, when the mantra was, "Whatever the doctor orders."

Today's patients are better informed about their options and anticipated results, and that is a good thing. But before we get carried away and assign all decision-making over to the patient, it is important to remember that healthcare is still a service provided by highly trained individuals. Unfortunately, even in the most skilled hands complications or unforeseen events can, and sometimes do, occur. And that is the subject of the next chapter.

12

Managing
Potential Complications

*Success is the ability to go from one
failure to another with no loss of enthusiasm.*
—Sir Winston Churchill

As we saw in the last chapter, while the successes accompanying the AGB in terms of the reduction or disappearance of chronic health problems is pretty impressive, any surgical procedure carries with it potential problems or complications. Although the incidence of these problems is generally outweighed by the benefits of the AGB, they must be recognized as real possibilities. That is the subject of this chapter.

Introduction

We have all seen actors dressed in surgical attire, playing the roles of surgeons, assistants, anesthesiologists, and nurses in dramatic operating room scenes. While some of what is presented is fairly accurate, much of what you see and hear is designed more for entertainment than anything else. Some of the newer health documentaries are a bit more realistic, and they often show an entire operation from start to finish. Even so, these procedures and the patients are often selected in advance for demonstration purposes, and you aren't likely to witness any major problems or complications.

Surgical complications and poor outcomes can and sometimes do occur. Within the surgical community a common statement is "The only surgeon who has never experienced a complication is one who has never done surgery." That is not to say that problems are inevitable for every patient, or even the majority of patients. Modern, minimally invasive surgery and anesthesia are generally much safer than a generation ago, but even so there are still risks, which are to a large degree dependant on individual patient factors. Obese patients with diabetes, high blood pressure, or cardiac problems are clearly at higher risk, but then again those are the very problems that lead to the need for bariatric surgery.

While it is important for patients to be aware of the potential risks of surgery, it is impossible to cover every risk and every situation with every patient. What you will find in the remainder of this chapter is just a brief explanation of some of the risks most commonly associated with the AGB. These problems can arise during surgery, postoperatively, and even long after the procedure.

Intraoperative Complications

When most people think of surgical risks, they immediately think of things such as uncontrolled bleeding or a heart attack, or something similarly catastrophic. But most intraoperative problems are less spectacular and are managed by the surgeon without incident. The key to minimizing problems during surgery is to recognize them before they become true complications.

Laparoscopic surgery has many well-recognized benefits, such as less pain, quicker recovery, and smaller scars, but it also has some limitations. Specifically, it can be more difficulty to identify certain unexpected injuries because the surgeon must rely solely on what he or she can see on the video monitor. Even so, experienced laparoscopic surgeons are able to identify and manage intraoperative problems with virtually the same capability as during open surgery.

There are some injuries that are unique to laparoscopic operations. When the surgeon inserts the laparoscopic canulas there is a chance of injury to blood vessels within the wall of the abdomen or one or more organs inside the abdomen. Injury to small blood vessels is typically not a major problem, but it may result in significant bruising around the site of the incision. Injuries of the intestine are uncommon, but they are a bit more likely in patients who have had previous abdominal surgery. Internal scarring, called adhesions, may cause the intestine to be stuck to the inside of the abdominal cavity. That not only increases the risk of injury to the intestine but also can make it more difficult to see such an injury. Such an injury could lead to a serious infection, but it may not become apparent for several days.

Electrocautery is a technique commonly used to control bleeding during surgery. During laparoscopic surgery there is a somewhat greater risk of unseen electrical injury to internal organs when electrocautery is used. These are particularly difficult injuries to identify because they can happen well away from the area the surgeon is looking at, and the damage may be virtually invisible. Once again, the effect of such an injury may not show up for several days. In the last several years, the mechanism behind electrocautery injuries has become better understood, and the incidence of such injuries has decreased.

When performing the AGB procedure the surgeon is required to perform a dissection around the area of the upper stomach and lower esophagus. During this process it is possible to injure either of those structures. The presence of an unrecognized hole in either the stomach or the esophagus is likely to become an extremely serious problem. If the injury occurs on the back side it can be nearly impossible to detect. Within about 24 hours the patient will generally develop a rapid heart rate, with fever and abdominal or chest pain. Should such signs occur after surgery, one or more tests can be used to identify whether the esophagus or stomach has actually sustained a perforation. If an injury is confirmed, the sooner it can be surgically repaired the better. The longer it remains untreated, the higher the risk of developing a life-threatening infection.

In addition to the esophagus and stomach, there are other organs and structures in the same general area that can be injured during surgery. The spleen is particularly at risk because it is very near the upper part of the stomach and is fairly easily damaged and can potentially cause major bleeding. Also, there are many major blood vessels in the same region. Fortunately, injuries of this nature are extremely rare during AGB surgery. But if major bleeding should occur, the surgeon very likely would need to open the abdomen to gain control of it.

Postoperative Complications

Postoperative chest pain, especially when accompanied by shortness of breath, could be a sign of a serious heart problem. The stress of anesthesia on the heart can be significant, especially for those patients with prior cardiac disease. That is one of many reasons why I feel that observation in the hospital for the first night is a good idea.

Following general anesthesia there are a number of respiratory problems that can occur. The most common respiratory complication is what is known as atelectasis. This occurs whenever you don't breathe deeply enough to fill your lungs completely. Small airways in the lower areas of the lungs tend to collapse, trapping mucus and bacteria in those tiny areas. This problem can generally be prevented if the patient will breathe deeply and cough regularly. If not, atelectasis can actually progress into pneumonia. Respiratory complications are more likely in patients who smoke or have pre-existing pulmonary conditions such as asthma, emphysema, and chronic obstructive pulmonary disease.

One of the most feared of postoperative complications is pulmonary embolus. This occurs when a blood clot develops in the veins of the legs or pelvis and breaks away, moving quickly through the heart and into the arteries of the lungs. If the clot is small it may result in only some transient shortness of breath and minor chest discomfort. But if the clot is large it can block one of the major arteries in the lungs. That not only blocks blood from passing through the lungs where it should be picking up oxygen and leaving off carbon dioxide but also puts tremendous stress on the heart. Pulmonary embolus can occur days, weeks, or even months after surgery, and it can be the cause of sudden death. Most blood clots begin while the patient is completely inactive while on the operating table or during the first few hours after surgery.

Normally the frequent contraction of the muscles in your leg acts like a pump, literally forcing blood through the veins. As long as blood is on the move it is unlikely to clot. During the total inactivity of anesthesia, as well as the limited muscular movements of the initial postoperative period, blood has a tendency to pool in the large veins of your legs and pelvis. If the pooled blood clots inside those veins, it may remain there until it dissolves, or become permanently affixed to the wall of the vein. The clotting of this pooled blood is known as deep vein thrombosis (DVT). But if the clot breaks free, it becomes a pulmonary embolus.

The best way to manage DVT and pulmonary embolus is to prevent the clot from forming in the first place. That is particularly true in bariatric surgery. As a group, obese patients are at greater risk than most normal-weight people for developing DVT during surgery. To help reduce the risk, patients are given heparin, a blood thinner, prior to surgery and usually for 12 to 24 hours afterward. This makes blood less prone to clotting inside the veins. At the same time, the patients' legs are wrapped with specially designed leggings called sequential compression devices (SCDs). These devices squeeze the legs periodically during the operation and in the postoperative period, simulating the pumping action of active leg muscles. The combination of heparin and SCDs reduces the risk of DVT substantially. In addition, the sooner the patient is up and around, the sooner blood flow will return to normal.

Problems following an Adjustment (Fill)

Most patients have an uneventful surgery and recovery. I have had a couple of patients who decided they could eat solid food earlier than was recommended, which caused them chest discomfort and some spitting up of the food they just ate. But most patients follow our recommendations carefully and have few if any problems—that is, until they have their first adjustment. Even then, the majority of patients are able to modify their eating behavior to deal with the restriction imposed by the band.

There are those, however, who really struggle with changing their eating habits. For patients who have trouble with solid foods after adjustment to the band, the result is unpleasant. While that is not in itself a complication of the AGB, if it is allowed to continue it can lead to other problems.

Every time you regurgitate food or fluids there is a risk that some of it will go into your trachea, or windpipe. This is called aspiration, and it can lead to episodes of severe coughing and even pneumonia. Patients are particularly prone to aspiration if they try to eat while lying down or if they lie down shortly after eating. While the problem can occasionally be due to the band's being excessively tight, most of the time it is simply because the patient is eating too fast, taking bites that are too large, not chewing adequately, or not stopping when they first feel the sensation of fullness. If the problem reaches the point of causing pneumonia, the solution is to take the fluid out of the band and leave it out for a few weeks. The process of gradually inflating the band can then be slowly started over.

Some patients are so enthusiastic about losing weight that they want the band tighter and tighter. When the restriction gets to a certain point, the only thing that will go down is liquids. Eventually it may be difficult even to get liquids through, and the patient will quickly become dehydrated. This is a potentially serious situation. Our bodies can go for extended periods without food, but only a few days without water. Whenever a patient tells me they can't keep anything down, including water, the band is too tight. The solution to this problem is to remove enough fluid from the band to allow liquids to pass through easily. The patient should be able to eat solid foods as well, provided they are "small bites, chewed well, and eaten slowly." (Sounds like a broken record, doesn't it?)

Problems with the Port

At the time of surgery, the injection port can be placed in a variety of locations. I prefer to put it along the left side of the patient's abdomen, close to one of the small incision sites used to place a laparoscopic canula. The port is sutured to the surface of the abdominal muscle layer to keep it from moving.

Despite this fixation process, it is possible over time for the sutures holding the port to break. If that happens, the port can actually flip over, which makes it impossible to access it with a needle in the usual way. Occasionally it may be possible to manually flip the port over, but that may require fluoroscopy (X-ray) to visualize it. More often than not, if the port flips over it is necessary to return to the operating room and surgically reposition and secure the port to the muscle.

The reason why some ports flip over is not well understood. It may be due to excessive tension on the sutures, or extreme stretching of the muscles that it is attached to. This happens relatively infrequently, though, and usually is fairly easy to resolve. I did have one patient whose port flipped and following the resuturing procedure he developed an infection around the port. In his case, a new port placed in a new location was ultimately required to resolve the infection.

It is also possible for the port to leak some of the saline after an adjustment. This is not likely if the proper needle is used, since the silicone core of the port typically seals itself completely when the needle is removed. A leak can occur even if the proper, noncoring needle is used or if any part of the port other than the silicone core is punctured. The port housing is hard plastic and cannot be damaged by a needle. But the stem of the port can be penetrated by the needle, and that part of the port will not seal itself, resulting in a slow leak.

One of the symptoms of a leak is that the restriction seems to decrease rather dramatically over just a few days. When the port is again accessed there is less fluid in it than anticipated. A leaking port needs to be replaced. This requires an outpatient surgical procedure, but it does not require the surgeon to re-enter the abdomen or replace the band.

On rare occasions, the tubing between the band and the port can become the site of fluid leaking out of the system. If this occurs, it may be that the connection between the two parts of the system simply came loose. To fix this requires a repeat laparoscopic operation to find the two separated ends and reconnect them. Again, the band would not need to be replaced.

If the balloon portion of the band that controls the size of the stomach opening leaks, the band becomes ineffective and must be replaced. The most likely explanations for a band leak are either an unrecognized tear or puncture of the balloon during placement or material fatigue, which can occur over time. Fortunately, this is a very unusual situation. To prevent faulty bands from being placed, each band is tested by the surgeon prior to insertion to help ensure that it doesn't leak.

Delayed Problems with the Band

The most common significant complication encountered with the AGB is slippage. This is a man-made device being placed around a God-made structure, and it doesn't always stay precisely where it was originally placed. Despite the fact that the stomach is sutured over the band, it is still possible for the band to slip. It is possible for the band to move upward onto the esophagus. But what typically happens, if the band is going to slip, is that it slips downward.

The term "slipped band" is often used to describe one of two situations that are similar but not really the same. A true "slip" occurs when the sutures holding the stomach over the band break or pull through and fail. This slip is most often caused by excessive overeating with progressive stretching of the upper pouch. If the band slips down on the stomach, the pouch will continue to stretch, allowing the patient to eat more, which further compounds the problem.

With a slipped band the most common complaint is heartburn. When the band is positioned properly, the amount of acid produced by the small stomach pouch above the band is negligible. As the band slides down, not only is the stomach pouch larger but the amount of acid produced above the band also increases. The band serves to block the flow of everything, including the stomach acid, so it refluxes up into the esophagus, causing heartburn. This particular symptom can generally be improved by using an acid-reducing medication, but ultimately the slipped band will need to be addressed.

If the surgeon suspects a slipped band, the first thing he or she is likely to do is order an upper GI X-ray to document the nature of the problem. The patient swallows some liquid barium contrast, allowing the anatomy of the esophagus, stomach, and band to be defined. The presence of a larger than normal upper stomach pouch is clear evidence that the band has slipped. If the slip seems relatively small, it may be managed by simply removing the fluid from the band and then slowly reinflating it. This may or may not work as a long-term solution, but it is usually worth trying because the other option is another operation.

Gastric herniation is another condition that is commonly lumped under the title of "slipped band," because the symptoms are similar. However, this problem doesn't actually involve any movement of the band. In a gastric herniation, a portion of the stomach from below the band pushes its way up through the band opening. This is a potentially more serious problem, because the portion of the stomach that is herniated through the band can have its blood supply choked off. That causes rather severe pain and if left untreated can even result in the death of that portion of the stomach, with catastrophic results.

The management of suspected gastric herniation includes first removal of all fluid from the band to minimize the tightness around the herniated part of the stomach. An upper GI X-ray is used to document the problem, but occasionally the barium contrast never makes it up into the herniated part of the stomach, so it may not show up on the X-ray. An endoscopy can be performed to look inside the stomach, but it may or may not provide additional information. Ultimately, if a gastric herniation is confirmed, or even strongly suspected, the patient will need to have a laparoscopic operation to fix the problem.

The actual operative management of either a slipped band or gastric herniation is dictated to some degree by what the surgeon finds at the time of surgery. In both cases the options may include resuturing the stomach over the band, repositioning the band, or totally removing the band and potentially performing a totally different bariatric procedure. If the band is simply removed, without any restriction the patient is very likely to regain most, if not all, of their weight back.

Virginia's Story

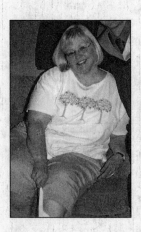 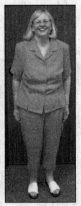

(Left) Virginia, pre-op, 242 pounds.

(Right) Virginia, two years post-op, 154 pounds.

Like most people, I tried all the diets. I weighed 242 pounds at 5 feet, 1 inch. I carried most of my weight from the waist down, but my face was puffy and my arms were big. I finally came to the conclusion that there was nothing left to try but surgery. I had a heart condition, Type 2 diabetes, my joints hurt, and I'd had breast cancer. In fact, I had a couple of other serious problems that had to be treated surgically, and I think they were all related to obesity, including the cancer.

In October of 2003, I got a band with Dr. Sewell. He'd done my mastectomy to treat the breast cancer, so when I started looking into the band and heard he was doing it, I didn't hesitate. Now, two years out, I've lost 88 pounds and weigh 154. The least I've ever weighed was 149.

I stopped taking my diabetes medication soon after the band surgery, and now I'm in remission. I also used to wheeze all the time, like I had asthma. My lung doctor said the breathing problems were due to my heart, which was weak due to chemotherapy. But, again, shortly after the band surgery, the wheezing stopped. To tell you the truth, I didn't expect to have the kind of results I had.

In the first six months, I lost 70 pounds. And it was very effortless. I found the more weight I lost, the more motivated I got. I was losing so fast, mentally I was feeling better and better. Exercise is extremely important even if it's not vigorous. I have walked from the beginning, every other day for a little over a mile. There's a high when you're first losing. But as the weight loss tapered off, little by little, I became more complacent. I forgot I was a fat person, and now I think of myself as a normal person.

I noticed I wasn't hungry at all for seven months after I got the band. Then I had kidney problems, and one had to be removed. The kidney surgeon said he had a hard time working around the port when he was trying to remove my kidney. But after I had my kidney out, I had a tremendous appetite. So I got another fill, and I think it was too tight.

I knew something was wrong when I had so much indigestion. I thought I had ulcers. I suffered all through the summer, slept sitting up, and finally came in for an X-ray, and it showed the band was slipped. Dr. Sewell put less fill in my band, and that's been better. I'm going to have to get the slip taken care of, and I'm scheduled for Dr. Sewell to go back in to reposition the band. I just haven't done it yet.

Anyway, I am sure I brought this on myself. I overate, then had too much retching. I know if the band is too tight or if I'm overeating, the throwing up can cause the band to slip.

For me, I know I have a disease that I have to manage the rest of my life. I can't say I'm not going to have diabetes tomorrow. That doesn't work. Even if it's in remission, like mine is now, I have to be aware and monitor my condition. It's that way with obesity, too.

I have a tendency to get discouraged until I look back at what I looked like before. I feel pretty good when I see those pictures. But after the kidney surgery when my band slipped, I gained a few pounds and I got really frustrated with myself. I started thinking déjà vu, here we go again, just like in the old diet days. But this is different. I've put on a few pounds, but I haven't gained all of it back plus 20 pounds, the way I used to. I'd like to be 125 to 135 pounds, but the reality is I'm going to learn to live with the 150s. And when I look at the old pictures, I'm happy with that.

Options If the Band Slips

While the problem of a "slipped band" can be managed successfully by repositioning and resuturing the same band, there is certainly some risk of having the same problem reoccur later on. Many surgeons ascribe to the old adage "Once burned, twice shy!" and recommend converting patients with slipped or herniated bands to a gastric bypass. Certainly this option should be discussed with the patient prior to any reoperation.

Another option that has shown merit in these cases is the removal of the band combined with a gastric sleeve resection. Unlike the gastric bypass, the gastric sleeve avoids the need to rearrange the small intestine. It is also solely a restrictive procedure much like the AGB, but without the band. However, a large portion of the stomach is removed under the theory that it produces hormones that lead the patient to feelings of hunger, so decreasing the stomach's overall size is likely to aid the patient in losing weight. This surgery avoids malabsorption problems because the digestive system is left intact.

One downside of the sleeve is that it can become stretched over time, leading to the ability to eat larger volumes again. Once it becomes stretched it cannot be adjusted or tightened like the band. Some patients relate that once they have had a problem with the band, they are less confident having a foreign object in their body, and the gastric sleeve provides a good alternative. The important thing to remember is there is no such thing as a perfect bariatric operation. No procedure comes with a guarantee. Any operation can fail, especially if the patient is unwilling to make the changes required in the way they eat.

Band Erosion

Perhaps the most serious complication related directly to the band is erosion. Over time the pressure of the band on the stomach wall can literally wear a hole in the wall of the stomach, allowing the stomach contents to leak out. If an ulcer develops in the lining of the stomach next to the band, it could potentially penetrate all the way through the wall of the stomach, creating a connection between the inside of the stomach and the band.

Generally band erosions occur months or even years after the band surgery and considerable scar tissue has already developed, which contains the stomach fluid to that area immediately around the band. However, the fluid is contaminated with bacteria, which cause an infection around the band. Patients with erosions usually complain of symptoms of fever, back pain, and even difficulty eating. But some patients have few if any symptoms from the erosion of their band, and may be totally unaware of the problem. Eventually the infection will make its way along the band tubing, and the patient will experience pain, redness, and swelling around their port. This is a "red flag" that strongly suggests an erosion has occurred.

An upper GI X-ray or an endoscopic examination will usually confirm the presence of an eroded band. If the band has truly eroded, there is no option except to remove the band. No matter how many antibiotics are administered, the infection will not resolve until the foreign object has been removed. It is not usually an option simply to repair the erosion and place another band. That is asking for trouble. It may be reasonable to perform either a gastric bypass or a gastric sleeve at the same time, depending on how inflamed the stomach is and whether the surgeon feels it is safe to perform any additional procedure.

Checklist: Signs/Symptoms to Watch For and Notify Your Surgeon About

✓ Swelling, pain, or redness in one or both legs
✓ Chest pain or shortness of breath
✓ Inability to keep down fluids
✓ Persistent heartburn
✓ Persistent vomiting or retching
✓ Pain, redness, or swelling at the injection port site

The exact reason why erosions occur is not known. Some surgeons have speculated that it is related to operative trauma to the outermost layer of stomach wall that occurred during surgery. Others suggest that it could be the result of ulcerations in the stomach lining at the site of the band caused by the pressure of the band or even anti-inflammatory medications that are known to cause ulcers. Either way, the risk of erosion is something that every potential AGB patient needs to be aware of. Fortunately, they occur in less than 1 percent of AGB patients.

Tracey's Story

I decided quickly, in just six days, to get a band back in 2003. It had to be removed a year ago, but I'm working on getting another band as soon as I can. Here's what happened.

I started at 357 pounds and I'm 5 feet, 1 inch tall, so my BMI was 67.5. I checked into the bypass, and at the time my insurance wouldn't cover it or a band. Since the band is so much less than a bypass, and it was even cheaper in Mexico, I decided to go down to Tijuana and get it done.

The first year I lost 96 pounds. Then my weight loss slowed way down.

First off I will say that my decision was very quick and I was not well informed. The worst thing for me was I did not have a local band doctor. I went back to Tijuana for my first fill, but I didn't keep up with the band in terms of getting regular fills, so I didn't continue to lose weight. I did finally find two band doctors in Oregon, where I live, who would do fills. But I didn't like one of them because I felt he wasn't very friendly and he was impatient, so I went with the other doctor.

I was going to get another fill, but then I found out I was pregnant. This was my fourth child and my fourth C-section. My obstetrician said he'd like me to have the fluid taken out of the band during the pregnancy, but I said as long as the baby is growing and isn't in any distress, I couldn't see any reason to remove the fluid. So we left the fill I had, and my baby is fine. And the C-section went without a hitch, too. The problems came afterward.

Two weeks after my C-section, in April 2005, my port got hot and swollen. On top of that, the band doc I was seeing left his practice. So I went to my primary care physician. She lanced the port area and drained the fluid built up there. The port site never healed. Looking back, I probably should have gone earlier to the other band doctor, the one I didn't like. But I waited and worked with my primary care physician.

From May 2005 to nearly December of 2005, I made regular visits to my primary care physician about the port site and took antibiotics. I wasn't in pain. I didn't have a fever. And I didn't notice any problems eating, like being able to eat less or being able to eat more. The port site stayed warm to the touch and a little swollen. I talked to my insurance about covering the replacement of the port. They said they would cover taking the port out to clean the infected area, but they wouldn't pay for a new port or to put it in.

Finally, in November, my primary care physician said that in her opinion there was something wrong with the port and I should find a band doctor. I felt my only choice was to go to that band doctor I didn't like. He was much friendlier the second time I saw him. Turns out the first time, he was having a really bad day.

He did an endoscopy and found the band had eroded through 60 percent of my esophagus. In other words, I had a band erosion. The only thing he could do was take out the band. Since it was life threatening, the insurance covered the removal surgery. It took from January to May for the port site to finally heal.

The scary thing about this for me is I didn't have a bunch of symptoms that indicated to me something more was wrong, other than what seemed to me to be a minor infection at my port site. I've met other band patients since, and within three or four months there were five of us that eroded— and we all had bands placed within a few months of each other. For me it had been two years, and I was fine until I had my C-section. Had I not gotten pregnant, I don't think I'd have had a problem, but I don't really know. The most fluid I had in my band was 1.5ccs in a 4cc band.

I've been without the band for a year. I had lost down to 248 before I had the erosion. I now weigh between 268 and 270. I'm hoping to get another band soon.

I wouldn't go back to Mexico. Prices in the U.S. for a band have come down to close to what it costs to go to Mexico anyway, when I include travel costs. Since I'm a self-pay patient, I cannot afford a gastric bypass. That is many times what a band costs.

I have an appointment to see about putting another band on. The concern now is that there could be too much scar tissue.

I will say I learned by having the band. I think a good psychologist could probably help me as well. I work at home, so I have access to food 24/7, and without the band I'm hungry all the time. With the band I wasn't hungry. I had moments when I wished I'd never got it. But now that I don't have the band, I wish I had it back. My hope is I'll be able to get another one, even though it will be funded out of my pocket again this second time around.

Band Intolerance

On numerous occasions I have had patients ask, "Can I have the band removed after I lose all my excess weight?" The answer is, "Only if you want to gain it back." For this reason virtually all patients have the AGB for life. Over time they learn to eat differently and don't really pay much attention to the band. In fact, most patients fear ever being without their band.

However, very rarely a patient will find they just can't tolerate the band. Despite having gone through the exhaustive assessments and counseling before surgery, once the band is in place they simply cannot tolerate the feeling of restriction. My approach to these patients is to work closely with them to achieve eating behavior changes before giving up on the band. More often than not the problem can be resolved. But when the patient becomes insistent, the solution may be removal of the band. While this is not truly a complication, it does represent a failure, and is obviously something we try to avoid through a careful pre-op selection process.

Handling a Crisis
G. Dick Miller, Psychologist

You feel you are in crisis. Something happens. You didn't expect it. You may feel fear or discomfort. Now is the time to use your new skills for rational thinking.

First question to ask yourself: Is it really a crisis? Another way to ask this question is: How big a problem is it? Do I have a chicken bone stuck in my throat? Or am I embarrassed because I'm getting up for the third time to go to the bathroom when I'm out at lunch with business colleagues? Which is a crisis? I can also ask myself, Would I call 911 for this? Or is it just inconvenient? If it's really a crisis, then it would be in my best interest to call in professional help quickly.

Some of us were raised or trained to "awfulize," "horriblize" and "catastrophize" things that go wrong in our lives. While it's understandable if we were raised that way, it doesn't help. We can't solve one crisis after another. If we elevate the inconvenient things in our lives into crisis after crisis, we simply wear ourselves out.

So if it's not a crisis, then it'll help my thinking and my well-being not to turn it into a catastrophe. I can call it what it is and then I can deal with it. By calling it what it is, I can decide what category it falls into. Here are five categories that problems can fall into: physical, social, emotional, financial, and spiritual.

Most people easily recognize the first four of these five categories. For example, going to the bathroom three times at a lunch is a physical problem and can also be categorized as a social problem. What I'm calling spiritual problems are those affecting my spirit or my core. I had a man in my band support group who didn't feel restriction with his band. In the beginning, he was upbeat and enthusiastic about his possibilities anyway. But as time went on, he got fills but felt no restriction. He saw other band patients lose weight when he didn't. And he got discouraged.

He started to identify with members of the group who had negative things to say about the band and what they couldn't eat. He started missing support group and then pretty soon stopped coming altogether. His problem was a spiritual one. He dropped out as his spirit, his motivation, and his belief in himself suffered. While spiritual problems tend to be underrated or even ignored, they are real problems.

Once you've defined which categories the problem fits into, that is the time to seek help. And the best place to find help for these problems is in your band support group. So many people try to solve problems on their own instead of taking the categorized problem to a group of people who can understand their situation and provide insight. There's no reason to go it alone, and it's usually not very successful.

In our example of leaving the table during a business lunch multiple times to go to the bathroom and throw up, a support group might suggest that you order something that goes down easily if you're going to talk, such as a bowl of soup. Or ask you to look at your bite sizes. Or you may find your band is too tight or too loose and you need an adjustment. (If the band is too loose, you can eat bigger bites sometimes but probably haven't learned to take small bites consistently.)

If you're not in a band support group, find one. You'll find the help and comfort you receive there will take you through a lot of problems before you're tempted to call them a crisis. And it'll help your spirit.

Checklist: Steps for Handling a Crisis

✓ Look at your thinking.
✓ Is it really a crisis? (Would I call 911?) Or have I awfulized, horriblized, and catastrophized it?
✓ If it's a crisis, call the appropriate professional for help.
✓ If it's not a crisis, what category does it fall into: physical, social,

emotional, financial, or spiritual? (Problems can fit into more than one category.)

✓ Now that you have your problem defined, seek help. Band support groups are a great place for this.

Poor Weight-loss Results

So what about those patients who simply fail to lose weight? These are not complications; they are simply patients who haven't achieved expectations. The issue of expectations is one that deserves some discussion here. From the surgeon's perspective, a good result is usually measured by improvement in obesity-related health problems. From a statistical standpoint most studies suggest that a good result is defined as the patient losing at least half of their excess body weight. But from the patient's perspective, a good result can be defined as almost anything. I have had patients who are excited just to have lost 20 pounds and kept it off for six months. Others who have lost 100 pounds or more still feel as though they have failed because they have 20 more to go to reach their initial goal.

As the famous saying goes, "Beauty is in the eye of the beholder." Results are determined by perspective. I learned some time back not to argue with a patient who seems satisfied with their results. However, there are many patients who are less than satisfied with their results. The reasons for dissatisfaction and poor results range from "I'm not losing fast enough" to "I expected to lose more" to "I thought it would be easier than this," or, my favorite, "No one told me I couldn't eat the things I like."

The most unfortunate thing that usually happens when patients perceive poor results is the return of feelings of self-doubt and poor self-image. Often these patients stop coming in for follow-up because they sense that their situation is hopeless. At the very time when they need help the most, they may give up on the program and sometimes on themselves.

I have had patients who stopped coming to see the dietitian, support group meetings, and our behavior modification programs for six months or a year at a time. When they finally come back to give it another try, it is amazing to see that their weight is almost exactly what it was the last time they were in the office. In other words, whatever weight they had lost previously had remained off. Once they get back into the program they typically start losing again, provided they have committed to changing their lifestyle.

For some patients the AGB just doesn't seem to work. I had one 340-pound man who had his band for about two years and lost a total of only 20 pounds.

His excuse was that he was too busy. He didn't have time to exercise. He didn't have time to come in for adjustments or dietary counseling. He certainly didn't have time for a support group of behavior modification sessions. In other words, he didn't have time to be successful. Eventually he went to another surgeon who removed the band and performed a gastric bypass. The last I heard he was losing weight as expected with the bypass, which is great. I can only hope that he will find a way to alter his lifestyle to ensure he keeps the weight off.

In the next chapter we will look at those critical lifestyle changes and the common hurdles and adjustments band patients face on their journey.

SECTION 5

Living with the AGB

13

The Emotional and Social Time Line

Aim for success, not perfection. Never give up your
right to be wrong, because then you will lose the ability
to learn new things and move forward with your life.
—Dr. David M. Burns

Just as there's a physical recovery period after surgery, there are periods of emotional and social adjustment that are pretty much universal for band patients. But, unlike tissue healing, which mends the surgical incisions, the time lines for psychological and interpersonal change are far less predictable. Throughout this book you have read over and over that weight-loss success after an AGB is not automatic; it requires a personal commitment to making lifestyle changes. But the reality is that there are numerous internal (psychological) and external (social) factors that continually challenge that personal commitment.

Also, just beneath the surface is a feeling of uncertainty regarding your new lifestyle and everything that goes along with it. Added into the equation for change are the social stigmas typically associated with obesity, not the least of which is your own concern that everyone else views bariatric surgery, and the AGB specifically, as a "last resort." This combination of influences invariably creates an underlying fear of failure.

Interestingly, there is another real problem that many obese patients have—that being the fear of success. If you've been overweight your entire life it can be frightening to consider what it might feel like not to stand out in a crowd. That concern is seldom talked about because everyone assumes that anyone who is morbidly obese wants to lose weight, and generally that's true. But I have seen patients struggle with their changing identity, and occasionally this can even lead to a subconscious sabotage behavior.

Success, like happiness, is a state of mind. I frequently use the example of results among professional golfers. Several years back I had the occasion to meet a young professional golfer who had actually won one of the lesser tour events a year or so before. When I asked how he thought he might do in the upcoming local event, he replied, "I hope to finish in the top 10." Had I asked Tiger Woods or Phil Mickelson the same question, I suspect the answer would have been, "I plan to win!" That is simply a reflection of confidence and attitude.

The really interesting part of this particular story is that later that same year the same young player who was hoping for success actually won the PGA championship, one of the four major events on the tour. From that point forward his career skyrocketed. He is currently ranked in the top 10 in the world. His swing didn't change. He doesn't hit the ball any farther. What changed was his level of confidence and perhaps, most important, a personal realization that it is okay to succeed.

Mike's Story

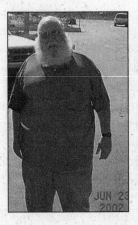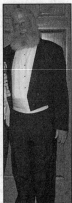

(Left) Mike, one year pre-op, 427 pounds.

(Right) Mike, three years post-op, 235 pounds.

I was 427 pounds, 6 feet, 3 inches tall, and 52 years old, and I was having trouble at work. I'm a land surveyor, and I was at the point where I couldn't get out of the truck and walk the 100 to 150 feet it took to help set up equipment. I ended up sitting, running my crew by radio. One day I heard one of them referring to my truck as "Mike's motorized wheelchair." That was enough.

I heard on the radio an advertisement for weight-loss surgery at Cedar Sinai in Los Angeles, pulled over, and called. I went in for the appointment, told the doctor my medical history, my weight problem history, and he did some tests. After about 30 minutes, the doctor said, "I think you need surgery, but I don't think bypass is for you." He asked if I'd considered the band. He spent an hour talking with me, sketched the band for me, and showed me how it works. I thought this sounded good. I started researching the band and quickly became convinced that it was for me.

I knew I was facing a life-threatening condition. I was on blood pressure medication, gout medication, and aspirin to thin my blood. I had arthritis in my knees, my left leg was completely numb from my hip to my knee, and I had a limp. I thought I could be dead in a year.

I tried insurance with no success. They refused four appeals including two done by an attorney who specializes in weight-loss claims for bariatric patients. I found a band support group and started attending. At each meeting I'd stand up and say I was still looking for a way to get the band but hadn't found one yet.

I am a professional Santa Claus, own my own costume, and at the holidays I offered my services to the band support group. After the gift exchange with the kids, a doctor who was visiting the group told one of the group leaders he wanted to give me a band. He was looking for a way to bolster his practice and hoped that word would get out that there was someone he'd been philanthropic to, and someone he thought was worthy who would do a good job with the band.

They thought he was kidding, so they didn't tell me. In April, at another support group meeting, the doctor came again to read a paper about the effects of weight loss on a person's self-esteem. At the time of the meeting in which we introduced ourselves, I gave my usual speech about fighting insurance. The doctor again asked the leader of the group to tell me he'd give me a band. They did, and I said to tell him I didn't have the money. He said you don't understand, tell him I will give him a band. Seven days later I was going in to have the band surgery.

I had started losing weight following the band rules, so I went from 427 to 385 in the year I was in the support group. I ate protein first, fruits and veggies second, then carbohydrates. And I took tiny bites, chewed 30 times before swallowing, and put my fork down between bites. I also became involved in Bandsters Yahoo group online, and during that year the owner gave me the group. When I took it over there were 4,000 members. Now it's the largest online support group in the world, with more than 10,000 members and 12 moderators. We don't censor, but we stomp on flames quickly, have no advertising, no spamming, and no fishing.

My band surgery went textbook perfect. It took 42 minutes. I had no nausea, no pain, and no soreness. I got up as soon as they removed the catheter, changed into my jogging suit, and walked the halls for about two hours before they made me go back to bed. I made sure I walked. I wasn't allowed to go back to my job for six weeks, so I made sure I got plenty of walking in. I was doing about 3 or 4 miles a day.

I'm still walking 3 to 4 miles a day, but not as exercise but as part of my job, since I can now be out with my survey crew. I walk all day long. I wore out a pair of boots in the last 18 months. I used to have trouble fitting behind the wheel of the truck. Now, no problem. I can carry 80 to 100 pounds of equipment over a hill and set up, and it doesn't bother me anymore. I'm glad I have a busy job.

In the first 18 months with the band I was losing 7 to 10 pounds a week, instead of the normal 2 or 3 pounds. I lost 218 pounds in that first 18 months, which put me at 212. And it was 100 percent the band that did it. I was very committed to sticking to the rules. No candy, no shakes, no ice cream (and that's one of my favorites—I consider myself an ice cream addict).

I notice running the bandster forum, that band people have to be some of the most impatient people in the world. I remember I lost 25 pounds between my surgery and my first fill. That's the time they call "Bandster Hell" because you spent all that money, went through all that pain, and now most people don't feel like much is happening. Some people don't even feel any restriction at all. I've decided that the bandster prayer is, "Lord, give me patience, and I want it right now."

I think people need education on nutrition. You need to know what a portion is, how much protein a serving is, and so on. And it's helpful to learn to put things together so you don't get bored, like how to fix chicken in new ways. The movie *Supersize Me* puts the spotlight on why we're getting overweight. Supersized portions are being presented as normal, but those portions are far from normal.

If you go to a website like fitday.com and put your parameters in, it'll tell you how many calories a day you require to live. Your basal metabolism is what you need to stay alive if you do nothing. Then they add your activity level and give you a result. If you don't have a nutritionist who can teach these things to you, then you have to learn yourself—a self-education process.

What most people need to do is control their diet around the proper nutrients and the proper quantities for health. Band patients need to know what their protein requirement is individually, not generically. I require 94 grams daily as a healthy, 6-foot, 4-inch active male, so the generic average of 60 grams daily won't be enough for me. The protein requirement is based on height, weight, gender, and activity level.

With the band, I found I'm not going to be permanently barred from eating something, but some foods take so much energy it's not worth it. For example, I don't eat stringy meat.

It's not that I'm never going to have cake again, but I had to get my mind wrapped around the concept that a portion is not a huge slice, it's a tiny piece. A normal portion is 3 to 4 ounces. So when I go to a steak house and they serve me a 16-ounce steak, that's four meals' worth. I used to eat two half-pound hamburgers. Now I eat what I want whenever I want, as much as the band will allow. Most of the time I do pay attention to my protein, my fruits and veggies, and I pay particular attention to getting enough water. Water is vitally important in the weight-loss process, and I work hard to get mine in each day.

I do exercise, but I've found that it doesn't have to be the social defini-tion. Exercise is moving mass through distance. The more mass you move (you are the mass), the more calories you'll burn. Exercise can be garden-ing, rowing a boat, climbing stairs, or walking the mall. It doesn't have to be organized in the gym or a formal workout session; it just has to be done.

I have hanging skin, but I'm not planning on having plastic surgery. I've been married to the same lady for 30 years, and I'm not interested in im-pressing anyone.

At 235 pounds, right now, I have gained back a little bit. But I'm also not being quite as strict with my dietary requirements. I went back up to 248, lost down to my current weight, and have maintained it for about a year and a half now. I now eat ice cream, a candy bar, even a milkshake, but the band controls me so I can't go nuts. Everything is in moderation. And I'm so glad to have it in there.

Your Psycho-Social Environment

It seems that almost everyone struggles with their weight, even those who don't appear to have a weight problem at all. Frequently you will hear someone who is only marginally overweight say, "I need to lose a few pounds. I think I'll try that new diet I just read about." Then they'll turn to you and ask, "Would you like to do it with me?" These are what I refer to as social dieters. They almost make dieting sound like fun, especially if "we" do it together. Virtually all mor-bidly obese people are surrounded by social dieters, many of whom are close friends or family. They mean well, but these folks have an entirely different per-spective on weight loss than someone who has fought a losing battle with their weight most of their life. That is why they can't understand why you can't lose all your weight on their diet.

People with serious weight problems don't want to join a dieting group where everyone else is trying to lose 10 pounds. They'll be the first to lose that much, but no one ever seems to notice. Unlike the social dieter, dieting for a morbidly obese person has always been a very lonely experience that invariably has ended in failure. Along with failure to successfully lose weight come the feel-ings of guilt and even shame. Once again those internally programmed behav-iors overrule reason and commitment. Is it any wonder that morbidly obese individuals are often emotionally stressed? Given this situation, the decision to have weight-loss surgery is often viewed by both the patient and those around them as one of desperation.

I have heard many patients say, "This just has to work," and in that statement is contained a tremendous amount of internal pressure to succeed. Family and friends are apt to say, "I know you can succeed this time if you'll just put your mind to it," further adding to the pressure to perform. You sense that everyone is watching you, and you silently wonder if the purpose of their observation is just to see you fail yet again. The irony is that all of this is usually occurring within the same psychological and social environment that helped lead to your obesity in the first place. Something clearly has to change! Your success may hinge on your ability either to change the environment around you (which is not likely) or to change the way you react to that environment. This doesn't happen overnight.

There is an obvious transitional period that occurs during the first few weeks after surgery when your old friend "food" has been taken away. One of the keys to a successful transition is finding something else to fill that need for comfort and gratification. For some this is a much bigger challenge than it is for others, but each and every band patient I have seen struggles with this issue to one degree or another. As you might expect, one of the most effective ways of learning to cope with this change is to become part of a group that actually understands your predicament, because they have been there.

To understand this psychosocial aspect of obesity surgery better, we must first acknowledge the impact that changing our eating habits has on our relationships with others. We are social creatures, and we are also social eaters. Eating is a very common group activity. In fact, it is one of the most basic of all social activities, and eating together has become a big part of our culture. Is it any wonder why most diets fail? Peer pressures associated with eating are simply too strong to resist. Some programs, such as Weight Watchers®, attempt to create a group dynamic in support of the act of dieting. Some are more successful than others, but ultimately all "diets" rely on individual willpower. Eating, on the other hand, takes on more of a herd mentality.

In contrast, surgery is by its very nature pretty much a solo proposition. It is also a totally passive activity. It's something that you have done to you, and it requires you to totally relinquish control—not a very comfortable situation. It has been my experience that many people feel better about having an operation if they know one or two other people who have had it or are going to have the same procedure, so they can "share the experience." Life's struggles are always easier when we have someone to share them with, right?

A number of interesting stories have either been written or documented in news reports about families or work groups who have all had band operations. The studies show that results tend to be better for everyone when done as a group. The latest in reality television has taken competitive weight loss to a whole new level. This is group dynamics in its truest form.

The promise of the band is that it will help control the amount you can eat and suppress your hunger. Unfortunately, it doesn't alter your desire to be part of the social scene. When you get into a situation in which everyone else is eating, and you are not able to participate the way you once did, you could feel left out, even though you are physically present. Many morbidly obese people have unintentionally advanced their disease by subconsciously building a circle of friends who are also overweight. They typically plan most of their social activities around the one thing at which they have always excelled—eating! Is it any surprise that once they have a band they start to feel like a social outcast?

Band patients have told me that their inner dialog in these situations goes something like this: "Everybody else is eating and enjoying themselves; why can't I? Here I sit eating my 'child's portion,' and everybody is looking at me like there's something wrong. They must think I don't like the food. Do they know about my band? Should I try to tell them? No, they'd just start asking how much weight I've lost, and I don't want to go there! Maybe next time I'll just stay home." This scenario is actually quite common, and occasionally I'll see an AGB patient that has become a self-imposed social recluse.

Isolation is extremely damaging to a band patient's psychological recovery. Being part of a group makes us feel more secure, and whenever we feel separated from our group security we become uncomfortable and even afraid. Why else would so many band patients report spending countless hours in Internet chat rooms? They need to feel the security of being part of a group. Feeling secure is a major key to your success, so get involved in a group of some sort that can help provide you with support as your confidence grows.

In my practice, we aggressively promote this by utilizing group sessions in almost every aspect of our comprehensive weight-management program. We take full advantage of the positive reinforcement that patients tend to provide each other. This includes group sessions with our dietitian, group sessions with our psychologist, and our monthly support group meetings.

Re-establishing Your Circle of Friends

It is totally illogical to suggest that in order to lose weight you must seek out a whole new group of "band" friends. If that were true, no one would ever succeed.

However, it is true that your success will depend in part on how supportive of your efforts those who are closest to you are. This can happen only if they understand the process you are going through. If those around you are constantly critical of your efforts, it's going to be extremely difficult for you to remain positive.

The fact is that the people around you really may not know what to say or how to act. This isn't because they don't care; it's because they simply don't know much about what you are going through. They can't relate. To avoid this you will need to take an active role in their education. One of the reasons we've written this book is to provide nonpatients with an explanation of what the AGB is and how it works. Even so, you must recognize that it may be very difficult for anyone who doesn't have a band to truly comprehend what you are going through.

Your closest friends may sometimes say the wrong thing at the wrong time. If they do, be quick to forgive them. It will help you both. It will also help you avoid the situation in which others are afraid to say anything because they don't want to offend you. Actively communicate with your friends. Let them know what's happening and how you feel about the changes you're making in your life. If you do, they will soon realize that you are still the same person you've always been; you just can't eat the way you used to. (By the way, that's a good thing.) Once they see your new positive attitude, it is quite likely that they'll be coming to you for advice on how they too might learn to better control their own eating habits.

Kim's Story

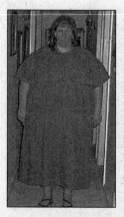 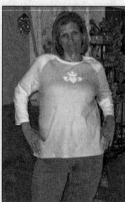

(Left) Kim, pre-op, 401 pounds.

(Right) Kim, four years post-op, 183 pounds.

I'd always been overweight. I was over 200 pounds in high school. But I got to the point where I weighed 401 pounds at 5 feet, 5 inches, so my BMI was 66.7. I was able to carry my weight, no problem, and I was always very active. But I decided that my weight was too much and I needed to do something drastic and started looking into surgery.

Like everyone else, I tried weight-loss programs. I'd lose a little, then put back on twice as much. Phen/Fen® was the most successful for me, but they took that off the market. At the time, I decided on a surgeon who was doing the duodenal switch (DS). It's more drastic than the RNY. My surgeon told me DS is for people in the "super obese" category only because they fear people with less of a problem will lose too much weight, since the surgery leaves the patient with less absorption capability than the gastric bypass. My insurance would pay for the DS, so I went for it.

After my DS surgery in 2003, I dropped 150 pounds within a year. I didn't put in a lot of effort and found it almost unbelievable how fast the weight came off. It was an easy, easy loss. But one thing the DS didn't teach me was how to eat. Then after about a year and a half, my weight loss stopped. Basically I went on with life, but at 250 pounds instead of 400 pounds.

When I came up with a blockage from adhesions wrapped around my intestines, I went back to my surgeon. He asked me about my weight loss and suggested the band. He'd stopped doing the DS by then and was doing only band surgeries. I found that my insurance would pay for all of the band with a $5,000 deductible.

I thought it was a good idea, so when my surgeon went in to repair the adhesions in January of 2006, he added a band. I'm now down to 183 and am still losing. I'd like to be about 140 pounds.

If I had to do it again, I'd do the band first. I didn't learn anything from having the DS. The band has taught me what to put in my mouth and to choose good food. If I make a mistake, the feeling of it getting stuck and throwing up is unpleasant enough to motivate me to change. It's like Pavlov's dogs. When that happens, I think, "I'm not going to keep doing this to myself." As a consequence, I've learned to make better choices and learned to eat slowly. It keeps me in check with much faster feedback. For example, if I want cake, I have some, but just a couple of bites. When I had only the DS, I would eat the whole piece of cake. In a while it would make me sick, and in a few hours give me diarrhea.

I also found that my body had compensated for my eating behavior after the DS. My surgeon told me when he went in the second time, to place the band, that my stomach had stretched out and was normal size again. I was anemic and malnourished before my band surgery, so I was in serious trouble health-wise and didn't know it. Now I'm still struggling with anemia, but I make sure I eat better. I also take iron and vitamins every day, which I didn't do before.

One thing I'm excited about is that I have a job I could have never had when I was 400 pounds. I work at a health spa as a youth services director. I exercise daily as part of my workday. This would never have happened three years ago. Back then I was director over a chain of preschool programs, so I was doing pretty well in life. But it's more fun now.

Give Yourself Support

All of this group stuff sounds great, but what about the rest of the time, those hours when you are alone? It is important to recognize that as you go through the personal changes demanded by the AGB you will frequently have to be your own support. To do so requires that you first take ownership of the process. In other words, make this "your" weight-loss program and take pride in what you are doing and in each goal achieved. You also must be completely honest with yourself.

I have seen patients who carry this self-support to the extreme. These are the ones who spend countless hours on the Internet, researching every little detail of the AGB. Each revelation received from cyberspace results in a modification of their approach, attempting to match what someone else said worked for them. Ultimately, this approach leads to the creation of a whole new set of excuses. Don't fall into that trap.

The best way to get started supporting yourself is to have a written plan, outlining your specific goals, your strengths, and your known weaknesses. In the business world there are countless statements about planning, such as "Plan your work and work your plan," and "Failing to plan is a plan to fail." But the one that I think is most true for supporting your weight-loss effort is "A plan that is not written down is no plan at all."

So write down your plan. You will also need to include the particular methods you intend to use to maximize positive areas of your life and minimize situations that present the greatest challenges. For example, if you know you have difficulty resisting chocolate, your written plan should list chocolate as a weakness, along with a plan to eliminate that temptation by not keeping it in your house. Likewise, if you own a dog and enjoy the dog's company, write that down as a strength and make walking the dog part of your plan for getting regular exercise.

As the weeks and months go by you will want to add to your plan as you identify newfound strengths and new challenges. You may even be able to move something that started out as weakness into the strength category, which can have a huge impact on your psychological growth. As you progress you may even feel comfortable sharing your plan and your successes with friends and family. Once you reach the point of being comfortable sharing your personal accomplishments with others, you will also have achieved significant social growth.

Dealing with Head Hunger

G. Dick Miller, Psychologist

Head hunger is a common term among people struggling with weight loss. It refers to a condition in which you think you need food but your body is not actually the one demanding energy. Something else is triggering you to respond with food.

I believe that anxiety is the number one issue with head hunger. What happens when you're anxious is that your body triggers the same gastrological response as when you're hungry. Enzymes get secreted in the stomach, so the feeling is the same as hunger. And hunger causes pain. What further reinforces this is that eating can make you feel better—you can mix those enzymes with food, and the pain goes away. So essentially, you've treated your anxiety with food.

There are several ways to handle head hunger. For example, you can dilute the enzymes in your stomach by sipping water. Another option is simply to wait it out, promise yourself 10 minutes before you take some other action, which is how long it takes for the enzymes to be reabsorbed. You can do exercises to calm yourself, such as walking around the block, working out, or doing a few stretches right where you are. You can also practice calming relaxation techniques such as slowing your breathing and letting your breaths come in and out from deep in your stomach instead of your chest. Or you might choose an area of your body and become aware of how it feels, such as the cloth against your skin on your right arm, or the way your left foot feels in your shoe. Another option is that you can simply tell yourself the feeling will pass. Or you can eat a little bit of something nutritious, instead of a substantial amount of anything, to feel better. Limit your intake and wait to see if you still feel hungry.

Being aware of the self, how you're feeling, is the biggest help. Personal honesty is the key. If you call it what it is, either stress or anxiety, then you've opened the door in your thinking to treat it in another way. Once you correctly identify the uncomfortable feeling, all of these options for treating anxiety become available to you. And this change in thinking allows you to make a better decision for yourself.

Checklist: Seven Ways to Handle Head Hunger

1. Take a sip of water.
2. Wait it out (about 10 minutes).
3. Exercise—walk, stretch, etc.
4. Concentrate on deep, slow breathing.
5. Focus on how various parts of your body feel, such as the clothing on your arm or your left foot in your shoe.
6. Tell yourself that the hungry feeling will pass.
7. Eat a little bit of something nutritious.

Change Your Daily Activities

Now that you are armed with your own plan, success is just a matter of time, right? Well, maybe. I don't mean to sound negative, but just a word of caution. Our society and our individual lives move at an incredibly fast pace. The "new-ness" of AGB surgery wears off rather quickly, and you'll soon find that nothing has really changed. The stresses of daily life are still there. Virtually everyone has a "to do" list, but rarely if ever are we able to get all the things on our list done. So, out of necessity we prioritize, focusing on those problems that repre-sent immediate needs, usually our job, our family, or a particular relationship.

However, we tend to procrastinate when it comes to our list of self-improve-ments. As we've discussed, many personal behaviors become more or less pro-grammed responses. The keys to unprogramming your responses are, first, make yourself, and in particular your health, a priority on your "to do" list, and second, embrace the idea of change. In the next chapter we will discuss how to implement these keys to changing your lifestyle.

14

The Lifestyle Change

I don't know the key to success,
but the key to failure is trying to please everybody.
—Bill Cosby

Changing your lifestyle is hard—really hard! I can't begin to tell you how many patients have said to me, "I'm too busy to exercise right now, but I'll get started as soon as my job settles down," or "I'll start eating better as soon as I get my family situation under control." Similarly, many patients have told me, "My job requires that I go out to dinner with clients. I can't just sit there when we're at a fancy restaurant."

Then there is the ultimate rationalization: "I'm going to Italy," or "I'm going on a cruise, so I need for you to take the fluid out of my band so I can eat." Does that sound the least bit logical for someone who has just undergone a surgical procedure to help them lose weight? The reality is that logic often has nothing to do with it. We are creatures of habit, and we don't like change, particularly when the comforts of our lifestyle are challenged.

Six Factors for Success with the Band (And IQ Is Not One of Them)
Steven Greer, Ph.D.

Since I had complete data for 83 patients over a two-year period, I decided I'd try to determine statistically if there were factors we could identify from the psychological testing to help us determine who has a better chance for success with the band. I took the top performers, those in the top half of the group in weight loss, and looked for common patterns or characteristics in that group from the psychological testing. What I found was an equation weighted for six factors that predicted the more successful patients.

First, I want to note that intelligence was not a factor, meaning that there was no strong relationship between the person's estimated IQ and their weight loss. So the good news is that you don't need to be brilliant to do this.

But there were six characteristics from the psychological testing that typified the people who did the best. One factor was being female. Overall, the women were more consistent losers over the two-year period than the men. Women outnumbered the men nearly three to one, which is pretty much what we see with weight-loss programs in general. I have noticed, looking at the numbers, that some of the men seemed to pick up their progress again in year three. My guess from looking at the data is that some of the men had a setback, made an adjustment, and did better in their third year.

The second factor was marital status. People who'd been separated, divorced, or widowed did better than those who'd been married their whole lives or who had never been married. My guess from this is that people who have navigated severe life changes, who have faced some adversity, face up to the demands of the band better.

Third, people who could admit to having some troubles, at least some emotional distress, did better at losing weight. I compared the data with my notes on the one-on-one interviews. The pattern I discovered was that those who seemed invulnerable, who were annoyed at doing psychological testing at all, and said their only problem was that they ate too much, didn't do as well with the band. The ones who could talk some about their problems, most of which were minor, did better in their weight loss. My belief is that the patients who were more willing to admit some vulnerability are more realistic about themselves, more open to receiving help and advice, and accordingly they did better. If you're a paragon of virtue and think you're going to conquer the world, then you probably won't do as well.

The fourth factor of people who did well was that they had lower scores on ego strength, meaning they could admit they had some problems coping. This goes along with the third factor, of being able to admit vulnerability.

People who produced certain psychological test scores suggesting less addictive potential did better with the band. By addictive potential, I mean those who tested as not as susceptible to addiction. I believe that addictive potential shows up in one of two ways. First, there are people who have a strong need for excitement in their lives, and those folks usually find their way to stimulants such as amphetamines.

Second, another whole set of folks feel a need to control negative emotions, especially depression and anxiety. As an example, these people might learn that heroin makes you feel really grand for a while or that alcohol can suppress emotion. So this group tends to adopt chemical substances that remove negative emotion, which for a while leaves them feeling pretty good. As we know, long-term, both of these solutions (for either excitement or controlling emotions) lead down paths that produce problems. But the significance for us, in looking at band patients, is that the people with less addictive potential were more likely to be top performers in their weight loss at the end of two years.

The final variable suggested that a tendency toward a personality that is aggressive, competitive, and more self-absorbed did better with the band. In personality clusters these are Cluster B personality types.

Let me explain. There are three personality clusters. In the extreme, Cluster A people are detached, aloof, and not involved with people. Cluster B types are aggressive, competitive, looking out for number one, self-interested, Type-A personalities. Cluster C personalities are anxious, worried about relationships, and what used to be called "neurotic." Those people who had Cluster B tendencies did better with their weight loss, perhaps because they were more comfortable looking out for themselves.

Let me say that this data is not intended to be absolute. These are just predictors, things we look for to assist us in helping band patients be more successful. This doesn't mean that if you have only some or none of these characteristics, you won't do great having a band.

In conclusion, you don't have to be brilliant to do well with the band. However, it helps if you've gone through some difficult situations and survived. It also helps if you have less of a tendency toward an addictive personality. It's helpful if you can admit you've got problems in your life and perhaps even that there are times when you've contributed to your weight problem. And finally, we found that those who are a little competitive, self-interested, more confident, and a little more aggressive did better.

Checklist: Characteristics of Top Weight-loss Performers with the AGB over a Two-year Period

The people who did best with the band included

- ✓ Women, who generally did better than men, especially initially.
- ✓ Those who had navigated severe personal distress in the past, such as divorce or widowhood.
- ✓ Those who could admit they face some emotional distress currently.
- ✓ People who could admit they didn't always cope well, meaning that they could admit they contributed in some way to their obesity.
- ✓ Those who tested with a lower potential for addiction.
- ✓ People who tended toward self-interest and more competitive types.

Transformation of Habits

Our lifestyle is composed of a combination of personal habits that we repeat day after day, week after week, and year after year. Going to work, going to lunch, watching television, even what time we go to bed, are all part of our lifestyle. For some, sedentary habits make up their entire lifestyle.

A habit can best be defined as a repeated behavior that has become more or less automatic. Some habits are good, like brushing your teeth. Others are not so good, like always cleaning your plate because your mother told you to, back when you were a child. And, as the old saying goes, "Old habits die hard." Lifestyle habits are particularly hard to break when they involve an overindulgence such as overeating, or any other comfortable activity, such as lounging on the proverbial couch. One of Newton's laws of physics states that "objects at rest tend to stay at rest." I'm sure you can relate, right? But, if you are going to succeed in achieving your weight-loss goals, you must make changes.

The best way to eliminate any old habit is to develop a new habit to take its place. That is precisely what happens to people when they stop smoking without their even being aware. We have all heard people: "As soon as I stopped smoking, I started gaining weight." You may have even experienced this phenomenon yourself. Some people convince themselves that when they gave up cigarettes, something happened to their body that caused them to gain weight for no other reason. Obviously, instead of putting a cigarette to their lips repeatedly throughout the day, they simply used the same habitual hand-to-mouth motion to put food into their mouth. One habit was simply exchanged for the other. Clearly, it doesn't make sense to go back to smoking as part of your effort to lose weight. There really is no "lesser" of those "two evils." The key is to find healthful habits to take the place of unhealthful ones.

Before any new behavior can actually become a habit, it must first be performed once, then repeated over and over. Just because you eat a fruit plate for lunch tomorrow doesn't mean you are going to have the same thing the next day, or next week. You may want it to become a habit, but it won't be until it becomes automatic.

It's a Thinking-Style Change
G. Dick Miller, Psychologist

I hear a lot about the band as a lifestyle change. And it is. But the best, most efficient way to start is with a thinking-style change. I believe that band patients have to start filling their lives with something else besides food, and that starts in their heads.

It's an incredible change when you think about it. I'd say 90 percent of the conversations I have with people I know are around food. We talk about how delicious it is, how much we "love" certain foods, what restaurants we're going to, and on and on. But for a band patient, that needs to change. And some band patients resent that, at least for a while.

But the truth is, we've had this unhealthy thing in our lives, this relationship with food, and it's important to fill our lives with something else. Mental health starts with honest thinking. Stop romanticizing food. Stop organizing your activities around eating. Stop using chow to deal with anxiety. And that starts in your head, with your thinking. The lifestyle change starts with accepting that it would be in your best interest to think differently about food.

We can teach ourselves to believe that food is not a solution to our problems. It's not love. It won't fix us. It was killing us. We don't have to say how much we "love" a dessert or that casserole is to "die for." Instead, we can start talking about food like the necessary fuel it is.

You don't have to change your thinking. You can get a band without working on your thinking and let the restriction attempt to change your behavior enough so you'll change your mind. But it's harder to do it that way because you'll end up dragging along your will and emotions. It's much easier to come into the band lifestyle reframing your thinking from the start.

For those of you who don't know, here's how reframing your thinking works. Let's say you're upset because you know you can't eat the donuts a coworker brought in to work one day. So maybe you find yourself thinking how deprived you feel. You can reframe those thoughts by saying to yourself, "You know, being able to eat all the donuts I wanted wasn't worth all the pain and suffering I felt." Remind yourself how it felt to wedge yourself into an airline seat or not be able to sit in a booth at a restaurant. Or think of your future, how great it will be not to have those extra pounds under your arms or around your middle.

If you do that, will you suddenly just feel better, all glowing and grateful? Not at first. There'll be some discomfort. It will be necessary for you to tolerate those uncomfortable feelings for a while. But they will pass. And overall, you'll have what you've really wanted all along—a healthier you, both mentally and physically.

Getting Your Body in Motion

New behaviors only come about as a result of new thoughts. "I think, therefore I am." Descartes penned those famous words nearly 500 years ago. It remains true today—in order to develop new lifestyle habits you must first change the way you think. Instead of finding reasons why you can't exercise, you need to search for opportunities to exercise. Rather than thinking about all the foods you can't eat, make a list of all the things you like that are nutritious and consistent with the restriction of your band. When your thoughts are negative, your actions will be as well. By thinking positively you will act positively. Results follow action and action follows thought.

Part of your changed thinking process should include setting definite goals for yourself: not just in terms of pounds to lose, but very specific new habits that you wish to develop. Your dietitian can help you outline a diet strategy that can be the foundation of your new eating habits. If one of your goals is to get more exercise, don't just run out and join an exercise gym with a plan to "work out" three days a week. Like many, you may never actually set foot inside the place. (Don't tell me! You've already done that? More than once? You're not alone.)

If your plan is to establish a new exercise habit, first practice the behavior of actually exercising, even if it is just walking around the block every day. Make the activity, not a membership, part of your lifestyle.

As you develop new healthful habits, you'll find many opportunities to expand them. Joining the gym may be one of those expanded efforts, but be realistic as you expand your goals. You are not going to become a marathon runner in the next six weeks. How do you think people who exercise two or three hours every day ever find the time? Are they just not as busy as you are? The fact is that somewhere along the line they made exercise a priority, they had the "thought." Then they performed the "behavior" repeatedly. Eventually it became a "habit" that is now automatic. Because their new habit was enjoyable, they gradually and excitedly increased the amount of time they devoted to it.

I know what you're thinking. "He makes that sound so simple. Doesn't he understand that I can't exercise? It hurts too much!" Well, here's the truth. Yes it hurts, but it isn't going to get any easier until you lighten your load. One good option is swimming or a water aerobic class. The buoyancy of the water substantially reduces the stress on your hips and knees. Just try it! At first it will feel awkward and even a little silly getting in a pool with a bunch of other overweight people, so start by changing the way you think about exercise. What do you have to lose, except the weight you've been struggling with most of your life?

"Threading In" Exercise
Julie Hillis, Exercise Physiologist

Everyone knows that exercise is important. I don't have any trouble selling that concept. But I'm not sure people always know why. One critical reason that exercise counts is that it is a hormone stimulant. One of those hormones stimulated is serotonin, which helps to counteract emotional blues and depression. In addition, serotonin improves the quality of sleep, and thus patients feel less fatigued.

What I see a lot of is patients being told to "just start walking." Well, if you're someone with bilateral osteoarthritis in your knees, which is a breaking down of the joints especially common in obese people, then walking is going to be hard. It is important to realize that a good exercise program should be completely individualized.

What I do is "thread in" the exercise program with the patient's life. What that means is we start slowly and design an individual program to promote success. Frankly, we know that if the patient isn't successful, they're not going to continue. We don't want someone to go out and do "boot camp" for four to six hours a day. We want a lifestyle change.

To start, we do a "current abilities" assessment by taking measurements of the patient's performance and body. As patients progress, the measurements provide important feedback. Change doesn't happen overnight. But in three or six months, when we reassess, people often say, "Wow, I remember it taking me 12 minutes to walk a quarter-mile, and now it takes me only 6." I also encourage patients to keep a pair of pants and shirt or blouse, so they can try those on at points as they are losing and really see their progress. That is an easy way to get some encouragement when you need it.

If someone is not exercising at all, I start them with three days a week. A lot of people will start out with only five minutes of continuous exercise. The important thing, especially in the beginning, is to get into an exercise routine. For most people who haven't exercised, this isn't going to be easy. But we want to start small and increase the amount of time spent exercising slowly, so as not to promote orthopedic or soft tissue problems. So the first 12 weeks are spent simply working into a regular schedule of exercise. Then every 12 weeks (three months) we "add on to the house."

As we progress in subsequent 12-week periods, we add abdominal and toning exercises. Toning is important because muscle (which is what gets built during toning) burns fat. And the more muscle someone has the higher their resting metabolism will be, which means that they'll burn more calories even when they're not moving.

What I love is for patients to work up to a minimum of 40 to 45 minutes of continuous movement in an exercise session. Our body's fuel tanks of glycogen and carbohydrates are the primary fuel sources that get burned in the first 30 minutes. So during that time, the body dips very little into the fat stores. But at about 30 minutes of continuous movement the body shifts into the aerobic state, in which it begins to use the fatty acids floating in the bloodstream as the primary fuel source. By the end of 45 minutes the percentage has shifted and the body is burning more fatty acids. That is an important point for patients to be aware of.

There is some disagreement, depending on what study you read, about when precisely the shift to burning fat occurs, but the critical concept to keep in mind is continuous, steady movement over time. Some people want to get on the treadmill and sprint for 10 minutes so they can say they've run a mile. However, they haven't achieved the goal, which is to get their body into that aerobic state so it's burning fat.

Checklist: Six Steps to Success for Your Exercise Program

1. Work with someone who knows what they're doing.
2. Start small. Build the habit of exercise first.
3. Remember, exercise makes you feel better. It acts as a hormone stimulant, helps counteract emotional blues and depression, and it can help you sleep better.
4. The minimum to build to is 30 minutes, three days a week, of continuous, steady movement. The optimum for fat burning is 45 to 60 minutes, three to four days a week, of continuous, steady movement.
5. Keep a pair of pants and a shirt or blouse that you wore before the surgery. Try these on when you've hit a weight plateau or just need some encouragement.
6. If you fall off the exercise wagon, go back to your exercise therapist anyway. Your body may have changed, and you may need a new set of goals. Plus, life happens to everyone, so don't get shamed into not going back. Progress happens when you stay with the program.

Some people can get to the point where they do 40 to 45 minutes of steady movement three to four days a week after the first 12 weeks. Others take longer to get there. The idea is to build in a way so there's not a lot of soreness associated with the exercise, and that's what a gradual build-up over 12 weeks will accomplish.

It may be that a patient can't get to their exercise goal because of other reasons, such as a bad hip, bad knee, or even being in a wheelchair. There are alternatives to a treadmill or walking, such as getting in a pool, bicycling, or even using an arm ergometer (a device that sits on a table and looks like bicycle pedals that you turn with your arms).

Building up to 45 to 60 minutes a day, three to four days a week, is the patient's investment in their long-term health. Even just 30 minutes a day, three days a week, is beneficial. After all, if you're willing to pay thousands of dollars for surgery, it makes sense to invest an hour and a half a week of your time in yourself.

I have noticed a pattern of behavior in band patients as I see them over time. I notice at their three-month follow-up they're in heaven, they're so excited about their progress and their weight loss. At the six-month follow-up they say, "I didn't lose as fast." So they're not as excited, until we measure and they see the inches that have come off. Between six to nine months, patients say to me, "If I don't lose another pound, I'm happy." They tell me they have more energy, they can go up and down stairs without trouble, but they do acknowledge that while the weight is coming off, it's more work now. At a year, it's not like their weight-loss program is over, but it is slowing down. But most people say to me that they love their new lifestyle and wouldn't change it.

There is no magic key to weight loss. It's calories in and calories out. But those who are exercising are toning up muscles and increasing their metabolism. The band is a tool to keep you successful, because you can't eat as much, even if there are days you want to. It's not like you have to give up everything you like. You can still have the foods you love, and it'll be okay. But the band is about making healthful choices, including regular exercise.

One thing to remember is to stick with your exercise therapist. This means going back even if you're not compliant with your exercises. I tell patients, "Don't get shamed into not coming back in here. Life is a roller-coaster. Sometimes you do really well, and other times you don't. Stay in the game."

As you're losing, there will be a number of physiological changes, and your therapist may decide to start you on something entirely new. For example, if you no longer require medication for high blood pressure, you may be safely able to do exercises that were previously not recommended.

The main message is stay committed. Your commitment to your exercise program will eventually yield rewards, even if you don't do it perfectly.

What's for Dinner?

In the last chapter we discussed the issue of eating as a social activity, but for many of us eating out has also become a primary source of nourishment. Many families eat out more often than they eat at home. Sometimes it's at a sit-down restaurant, other times it's drive-through, and of course there is the always-available home delivery. The constant is that someone else cooks it, and either they do the clean-up at the restaurant or we toss the paper and plastic in the trash. How convenient!

The restaurant industry has been booming for several decades because it saves us both time and effort. We can eat what we want, when we want, without having to go buy the groceries, prepare the meal, or wash the dishes. And everybody in the family can have something different. What could be better? Maybe if it were free! While prepared food isn't exactly free, at some places you can get more than enough calories to meet your body's needs for little more than the spare change in your pocket.

Sit-down restaurants are obviously a little more expensive because of the services they offer. To make up for this higher cost, some places offer huge portions. The food is actually fairly inexpensive to prepare, so it doesn't cost them much more to ensure that no one goes home hungry. It's almost comical when the waiter comes to your table and asks, "Anyone save room for dessert?" Despite the fact that you're "stuffed," the sound of homemade pie with ice cream can be hard to pass up. The temptation can become simply irresistible if they bring out that tray of sweets, so you can actually see them.

Well, the reason for this description of modern American dining habits is to emphasize the need for change. The main reason why most people become obese is simply overeating. Now you've got the band to help you eat less, but you can't expect to lose weight unless you actually do eat less. That requires a change in eating habits, starting with where and how you get your food.

Now, I know what you are thinking. "This guy is crazy if he thinks I'm going to start cooking three meals a day at home. I don't have time. Besides, the rest of my family won't stand for it." I agree, it is unreasonable to suggest that we return to the lifestyle of the 1950s, when mom cooked breakfast for everyone, prepared their lunch boxes, and had a hot meal waiting when they came home from work and school. But at the same time, it is totally illogical to assume success with the AGB unless you make some changes to your current eating habits.

While eating at home more often may be a good place to start, it won't really make a difference unless it also includes preparing healthful, nutritious meals in reasonable quantities. This implies that infamous word: "diet." But, I'm not talking about the painful depravation of the numerous diets you have previously endured. Instead, you need to develop a new, rational, preplanned eating behavior that is consistent with the restrictive nature of your band. This starts at the grocery store. Map out a meal plan for the week and buy only those things you need to prepare the meals you have planned.

If you don't have a plan for what you intend to eat when you go to the store, you will wander down every aisle, picking up all the same junk you've always bought. This will include chips, cookies, candy, and everything else that goes down easily despite the band. You will have sabotaged your weight-loss efforts before you even get the groceries to the car. Understand, if you buy snacks and comfort foods—you will eat them. It's that simple. Why would you do that, you ask? Habit!

I've had several patients tell me that they buy snack foods and sodas, but they are just for their family. One woman even told me that her son wouldn't stay around the house unless there were snacks available. While this may sound ridiculous to some, for others it represents one more unexpected obstacle to be overcome. You need to sit down with everyone in the family and explain that the snack foods and soft drinks they have come to expect are a thing of the past. They are being replaced by fresh fruit and low-calorie drinks.

No doubt there will be grumbling and moaning, but ultimately you and everyone in your family will develop better eating habits. So, how do you pull this off? First you must recognize the need (develop the thought), then be the instrument of change by initiating a new household policy (introduce the behavior). Only then will you be able to sustain it on your own behalf (the habit).

Supersize Me, directed by and starring Morgan Spurlock

This Oscar-nominated documentary is about American fast food and its effects on everything from elementary school children to legislation. In it, filmmaker Morgan Spurlock lives on nothing but McDonald's food for an entire month, with three simple rules:

1. No options: he could eat only what was available over the counter (water included!).
2. No supersizing unless offered.
3. No excuses: he had to eat every item on the menu at least once.

Spurlock received the award for Best Director at the Sundance Film Festival in 2004, and the film has received a number of accolades since.

Roseann's Story

I'm 50 years old, and my first 50 years were spent destroying my body. I didn't think it was fair to me or my husband that I couldn't be what we both wanted me to be. I tried diets, like Weight Watchers®, and lost and regained a lot of weight.

I'm a nurse, but that had nothing to do with my decision to get the band. I heard about gastric bypass, and it scared me. I went on a trip with another band person, and she told me about the band. I started looking up more information on the Internet. I knew I had to do something.

Within a month after meeting Dr. Sewell, I decided that he was going to be my doctor. I also decided to become responsible for my actions from then on. I knew the weight loss would be slow, but I didn't care how long it took me. I have to work for every pound of it, but that's okay.

I also knew my insurance wouldn't cover it. My husband said, "I'm behind you one thousand percent. Give me the checkbook. This is your new car." I think I might be a little more lax with my care if I hadn't had to pay for it myself. But since I did, I've been extra careful.

I had my surgery in April of 2004, and so far I've lost 64 pounds. I'm 5 feet, 2 inches and weigh 187 now. My goal weight is 132. That's 50 more pounds to go, but it doesn't sound like so much now. People around me say I should not have that much more to lose, but I assure them I do.

I remember Dr. Sewell saying when I went for a fill, "Some people just don't get it." Honestly, it took me about eight months to "get it." I would argue nonstop, saying things like, "I'm not losing," "I can't tell when I'm full," "Something is wrong here." He said I wasn't patient with the process. And then, about two and a half months ago, I got it. I realized it really was the portion size, and I had to trade food for exercise.

Exercise got easier and more manageable as I've lost. Now I enjoy jumping out of bed, doing my workout, and moving on with my day. I can do an hour to an hour and a half, but our dietitian advised me not to exercise seven days a week. She said that she doesn't exercise that much. I was so afraid that if I didn't go all seven days, I wouldn't lose the weight. There was still that fear factor.

I feel normal now. I'm acting like real people do. I was on blood pressure medication, and I'm off as of September 2004. I never had reflux again after the band surgery, but I waited to go off the medicine until September, too. I was prediabetic and now I'm fine. I had sleep apnea, tried the machine, then had airway surgery, but that didn't help either. I went through a lot of hell and pain for nothing. I still wake up sometimes in the night, but I don't have a real problem.

Some days are better than others. I have days when I can eat what seems to me like a lot and others when I can hardly eat anything. But overall this is a lot easier than being fat ever was.

Sometimes people ask me about my weight loss. When I tell them, they ask, "In how long?" Like it's a race or something. So I say, "I'll tell you how long it took, but it really doesn't matter because it's not a contest. I'll never go back to where I was."

Eating Out

Okay! You're not going to eat at home every meal, that's obvious. Going out to eat will continue to be something you do with family and friends. The key then becomes developing a strategy for eating out that helps ensure your weight-loss success and allows you to continue to enjoy this important group activity. You need an "eating out plan."

It isn't enough to assume that the band will control your portion size. Ultimately, that is your responsibility. At most restaurants the server will bring you more than you can eat. But I don't have to tell you that once it's in front of you, it can be hard to make yourself stop eating, even when you're full. Your "battle plan," and I mean that literally, should consist of several specific strategies that will make going out to dinner much easier.

One of the easiest ways to control your portion size is to share a meal. Before you decide where you are going out to eat or where you are going to order your meal from, get together with your spouse or your friend or whoever you are planning to eat with, and agree to share a meal. At the restaurant, order only one meal and an empty plate. When the food arrives, take a small portion for yourself and let the other person keep the rest. Don't let the server divide it for you; they will likely split it evenly, which may be too much for you and not enough for the other person.

Also, don't ask them to divide it for you back in the kitchen. Remember, part of the restaurant's strategy is to make sure you have plenty. They want you to come back, so they are likely to add a little extra to each plate. That's not what you need.

Depending on the restaurant, you may be better off ordering an appetizer rather than a full meal. Some restaurants even offer appetizer portions of most of their entrees, if you ask. Not only are the portions smaller, but they are generally much less expensive. If all you are going to have is the appetizer as your meal, have them bring it at the same time they bring everyone's appetizer or first course. You don't want those around you to feel uncomfortable eating while you are just watching. With your new eating style (slow down, small bites, chew well), it is likely to take you about the same amount of time to eat that appetizer-size portion as it will everyone else to eat their entire meal. So don't rush through it.

Another good option is to order off the child's menu. Some restaurants frown on this because they think you are just being cheap. They may even say that you can't order one of those items unless you are 12 years old. To address this problem I give each of my patients a small doctor-directed "portion card" that the patient can show to the server, or manager if necessary. Should the restaurant continue to refuse you the option of ordering off the child's menu, just remind them who is paying the bill and offer to take your business elsewhere next time. As I said, this is a "battle plan."

Sometimes you just don't want to share a meal, or you don't see any appetizers that sound appetizing, and the stuff on the child's menu is, well, "kid's stuff." Go ahead and order what you want, eat what you want, and take the rest home. But here's the trick. Tell your server that you want him or her to bring out only half of the meal. Ask them to box up the other half. Having less on your plate will help you avoid the temptation to overeat, and the food you take home will look more presentable when you get it home than if you scrape it off your plate into a "doggy bag."

While desserts are typically higher in calories than most other foods, that is not always the case. Again, sharing a dessert can allow you to sample a piece without eating the whole pie. It's all right to allow yourself a treat every now and then. Just don't do it repeatedly, and it won't become a habit.

There is one more important strategy that you will need to employ whenever you eat out at a restaurant. One of the jobs of the server when you first sit down is to bring you something to drink. Throughout the meal they will make sure your glass is always full, whether it is water, or tea, or whatever. But remember, with the band you are not to drink and eat at the same time. You can, and should, drink fluids as much as you like until your food arrives; then you need to stop drinking. Otherwise you'll eat too much. Drinking and eating at the same time is something you have done your entire life. It's a habit. Breaking that habit is not easy, especially when there is a full glass right in front of you. You'll pick it up and take a drink without even realizing it. The next thing you know they'll be right there, filling it up again.

Especially early on, you're going to need help to avoid drinking with your meals. One option is simply to ask the server to take your glass away when your food arrives. He or she is not likely to understand why, so you'll be asked whether there is something wrong. If this situation makes you uncomfortable, you can just leave the glass on the table, but you may need help remembering not to pick it up. Try this. Place a small napkin or even a bread plate on top of the glass as a reminder. This may sound silly, but it works. You will not be able to drink out of the glass unless you first remove the object that you placed on top of it.

This additional step will help you avoid the automatic behavior of drinking between bites of food. Any object on top of your glass will also send a clear signal to that guy who keeps coming around asking, "More tea?" Once you have mastered the technique of separating liquids and solids, it will become an established habit and you won't need any reminders.

No matter how careful you are to eat slowly, take small bites, and chew thoroughly, everyone has problems occasionally with overeating. It may happen that the food you just swallowed is not going down. In fact, it is causing considerable discomfort as your esophagus pushes harder and harder to force it down. You become convinced that it's not going down, it's coming back up. Certainly this can be a problem at home, but it is more of a problem when you go out to eat.

I had one patient tell me that every time she goes anywhere to eat, the first thing she does is locate the bathroom. She knows that at some point during the meal she will need to excuse herself and quickly make her way there to bring up what she just swallowed. Some patients face this situation at virtually every meal and just accept it as part of their new lifestyle.

Eating doesn't have to be that way. If this is happening regularly, one of two things is going on. Either the band is truly too tight and needs to be loosened, or you are still taking bites that are too big or not chewed adequately, or you are consuming food too fast. Spitting up your food should be a signal that something needs to change.

Patients tell me that they avoid spitting up by just ordering soup. They do this to avoid embarrassment, but that is not the best way to handle the situation. If you are spitting up all the time, and losing more than a couple of pounds a week, the band is probably too tight. But most people who come in complaining of spitting up at nearly every meal are often not losing any weight at all. Their food is going through the band; it just can't go through as fast as they are putting it in, or they swallow bits of food that are too large and the bites get stuck.

Checklist: Tips for Successful Eating Out

- ✓ Share a meal.
- ✓ Consider ordering an appetizer or off the children's portion of the menu.
- ✓ If you order a regular meal, ask the server to box up half of your meal in the kitchen to take home. The meal will look more appetizing for later, and you won't be tempted to eat too much.
- ✓ Follow Dr. Sewell's Golden Rules for AGB Patients on page 140.
- ✓ To avoid drinking with a meal, ask your server to take away your water glass when your food arrives. If that's not practical, place your napkin or bread plate over the glass. That way you can retrain yourself not to drink unconsciously out of habit during your meal.
- ✓ If you're struggling with eating out, find another band patient who is doing well and eat out with them. Watch how they conduct themselves during a meal.

One strategy that you may want to try in your quest to learn new eating habits is to go out to lunch or dinner with another AGB patient who seems to be achieving significant weight loss. With that idea in mind, we actually offer a mentoring program to our patients even before they have their surgery. If you don't know any band patients, the best way to get acquainted is through a support group. The experience of eating out together will not only benefit you as you watch how the other person eats; it will also serve to reinforce the behavior of the mentor.

Increasing Your Metabolism
Kirk Evans, Exercise Physiologist

I find, working with band patients, that they now have a tool they can use to help them with their eating style. What I mean is that the band helps them control their appetite and their quantity of food. However, the band doesn't control their exercise or their quality of food choices, and that's what I'm trying to get people to do.

What I find is that many band patients have never exercised. I try to get the patient to become aware of why it's important to exercise. One of the things I emphasize is weight training to maintain muscle mass and to help people keep their metabolism up. Most weight-loss patients have experienced losing weight on a diet, then have gained back more than they lost. The reason they gain back more, and put it on quickly, is that their metabolism is slower.

An especially useful tool I have to aid patients is a scale that allows me to do a body composition analysis. The scale sends an electrical signal through the patient and makes a composition diagnosis of the fat mass and the fat-free mass in the patient's body. (The fat-free mass is made up of muscle and water.)

This is useful because if you get on your scale at home, you'll see that you've lost 10 pounds, but you don't know if it's 10 pounds of fat, water, or muscle. With this scale you know what you've lost.

Another plus is that you might get on your scale after working out the way you've committed to and find that you've lost nothing. That can be discouraging. But using this scale, I may be able to see that you lost 2 pounds of adipose tissue (fat) and gained 1 pound of muscle and 1 pound of water. So this provides us with another way to measure progress.

While the band offers a more gradual weight loss than other surgical options, it's still a pretty drastic procedure. You're immediately going to reduce your calorie count. And your body needs to make a choice if it's going to burn fat or muscle to replace the food you're not taking in. As I've mentioned, I stress the importance of weight training so the patients can maintain their muscle mass and not suffer setbacks in that realm. I encourage the use of free weights or body resistance. For example, if people haven't exercised before, they might start with what we call chair stands—just getting in and out of a chair over and over. These exercises, while they sound simple, initially allow the use of the patient's own body weight to build up resistance.

My advice is to get out of the negative cycle. Exercise can be enjoyable and is obviously beneficial. I try to stress the importance of the overall health aspect of it. People can be thinner but not healthier. Patients who commit to exercise enjoy even the simple things, such as the ability to walk longer without shortness of breath and with less joint pain. They find that they can do things they either haven't been able to do in a long time or were never able to do. Overall, they become stronger and more conditioned individuals—both thinner and healthier.

Obesity Is Expensive; Thinner Is Cheaper

Whatever your lifestyle, it comes with a price tag. That's obvious. But are you aware of how high that price actually is? Being extremely overweight is expensive. The cost of food alone can be substantial if you have been eating twice as much as you need or more. I had one man tell me that he would routinely eat six chicken breasts at one meal!

Extra-large clothing also costs more, especially when you get into business suits and nice dresses. It is not uncommon for "plus size" garments to cost two or three times more than standard sizes. Transportation costs can also be substantially higher. Inexpensive compact cars may not even be an option if you're too big to fit behind the wheel. Coach class airline seats may not fit either, forcing you either to buy two seats in coach or to pay extra to sit in first class.

The point is that there are many day-to-day expenses that are higher because you are obese. Add in the cost of medications for diabetes, high blood pressure, high cholesterol, and other problems, and the cost of "living large" goes even higher. What about doctor visits and other medical treatments? If this is you, I don't have to explain the financial stresses of obesity. But the good news is that with weight loss comes substantial savings.

One patient kept a very comprehensive log of his living expenses, both before and after his band. Within four months of his surgery his average cost of living was down $440.00 a month. Other patients have shared similar results and are shocked at how much less they spend on food and medications alone. The clothing issue tends to be a two-edged sword. As you lose weight you are able to buy much less expensive clothes. You'll get really excited the first time you buy something off the department store sale rack. But at the same time, even sale items can add up if you are replacing an entire wardrobe. I urge my patients not to buy too many clothes the first time they drop a couple of sizes, because as they continue to lose, the new clothes probably won't fit in a few more months.

The fact that you are thinner will continue to pay financial benefits over the remainder of your life. That can be an important motivator to stay "on the band wagon." Try keeping your own log of your monthly expenses, and you will be amazed by how much money you have "left on your plate."

Linda M.'s Story

At the end of 2004 I talked to my doctor about a bypass, but he said he wouldn't recommend it. I weighed 249 and I'm 5 feet tall. Dr. Sewell was recommended by a friend and I went to his seminar, then decided to have the band surgery.

I lost 17 pounds on the pre-op diet, and I found it to be very difficult. But I had no problems with the surgery, though Dr. Sewell kept me overnight, anyway. He does that with everyone. But I had no restriction at all after the surgery. I got my first fill at six weeks, and I had very little restriction then.

The problems for me are not particularly eating. I've never thrown up food. If something gets stuck, I notice that I get a buildup of saliva and that usually has to come up. I've found that I have more trouble eating earlier in the day, so while breakfast is my favorite meal, I now have it at lunch.

I have reached a plateau and that's difficult, but my goal was to improve my health, and that's happened. My plan is to get another fill. I've lost 58 pounds, so I'm at 191. I had diabetes, and I'm taking only one medicine for that now at a 15 mg dosage and expect to be off it soon. I was taking 500 mg three times a day. I was also taking medication for high blood pressure and for acid reflux, and I'm not doing that anymore.

The band has also saved me money. I'm self-employed and was in a high-risk pool for health insurance in Texas that cost me $725 a month with a $1,000 deductible. Now I'm on a major medical and drug plan that costs $325 a month because I'm no longer considered high risk.

I'm a therapist, and I have a patient who had the band surgery with another doctor, who was in her healthcare network. But she's had problems because her port didn't heal for six months, and she couldn't get a fill. So she lost six months of weight loss. I have another patient who had a bypass and she's thin, and I mean thin, but she's been sick a lot.

One of the things I like about Dr. Sewell's plan is the comprehensive program, with the support group and the exercise therapist. I was over 9 minutes in the beginning on a quarter-mile, and after six months my quarter-mile was 4 minutes, 15 seconds. I got a treadmill after the surgery and joined Curves.

The other thing, and this is just me, but I'm a psychotherapist, so I think it's a good thing they have the psychological component. I didn't have to do that. I already have that training. But I know it's needed.

I met someone who had a bypass because that's all her insurance will pay for. This woman still wears long T-shirts and baggy clothes, even though she's thin now. That's a mindset problem. She still dresses as though she's heavy. She went to a doctor who doesn't have a comprehensive program. She did some support group online, but it's not the same.

It's my opinion that you shouldn't get a band if you think it's going to change your self-esteem or make you like yourself. You need to have that going in. Health is the best benefit, not vanity. Will looking better improve your self-esteem? Yes. But it's good to have that psychological component of the program to help people who are going to be disappointed or still struggle with their self-esteem.

I believe I'm going to want plastic surgery. I am in a size 16, and I can't get myself in a size 14 because of the apron of hanging skin from my stomach. I also want to have my arms done. In order to have the plastic surgery I will have to pay for myself, so I need to earn some more money. The plastic surgeon's office did tell me I could finance it.

Oddly enough, I won the money to finance my band surgery in Las Vegas while at a conference. And it was the exact amount I needed. I decided then it was meant to be.

If you do what you're supposed to, the band works. I like it that I can eat whatever I want, just not much, but that small amount is enough. No one needs to eat as much as they give you in a restaurant anyway. The people in China are not going to benefit from me finishing my plate. I like the idea that I can take food home and have two more meals. I had to work to find something I could eat in the morning, and now I eat protein bars. Overall, I like it that I don't have to struggle anymore. It's just easier. I don't have to think about what I'm going to eat and what I'm not going to eat. My life is not an ordeal. And it was before.

Your Image

We have spent considerable time discussing how to change your lifestyle and how you will benefit from it. We've listed many of the things that are likely to happen to you. But, how are you going to feel about these changes in your life? How will you respond to your new life? How are you supposed to deal with this new person you have become?

These are difficult questions to answer, because every person reacts differently. Some people embrace their new life with excitement and enthusiasm. Others are fearful of the unknown and tend to remain pessimistic, even after they have tasted success. Some patients have a very difficult time ever seeing themselves as anything but a "fat" man or woman. That is why it's important for you to participate in a support group or a psychological improvement program to help you develop a true sense of who you really are.

When it comes right down to it, you probably won't know how you will react until you actually begin to experience significant weight loss. Physically, almost everyone relates that they have more energy. I had a patient recently tell me that she has so much more energy now that she needs only about 6 hours of sleep each night, instead of the 8 to 10 hours she used to require. She's up and ready to go at 5:00 A.M. every morning and is far more productive throughout the day. While that's a bit more energy than most people have, it's an example of just how much natural vitality obesity can rob you of.

Having more energy affects every aspect of your life, from your job to your family life, your ability to exercise, and yes, even your sex life. Perhaps most important, when you have more energy other people see it and respond positively to you. Those around you will feed off your energy, making you a valuable part of virtually any situation. The natural progression then includes increasing self-confidence and a feeling of self-worth.

Another aspect of change comes in how people treat you. Anyone who is morbidly obese knows the reality of "obesity bias," especially in the workplace. Employment opportunities can be limited, and advancement may be blocked by those who perceive obese individuals as lazy or even less intelligent. But part of the problem may also be related to how obese people perceive and project themselves. Losing weight certainly changes your appearance, but for many the most important change is in their self-confidence. And it is this change that tends to open doors and eliminates ceilings in the workplace.

I have one patient who was very quiet and reserved prior to her band surgery. She had worked at the same job for several years and would never consider asking for a promotion or a raise for fear of being turned down. Within about four months of her band operation she lost around 40 pounds and her personality changed dramatically. She became far more self-confident and self-assured. She sought out a new job where she quickly became a much more visible contributor. Within a few months she was discovered by another company and was hired away with a new salary that was three times what she had been making less than a year earlier. Same woman—different attitude.

Other patients have shared similar experiences, and in each situation the story revolves around self-image. Virtually every self-help book ever written is based on the principles of self-confidence, self-motivation, and self-reliance. If you have perceived yourself as a failure because of your inability to lose weight, those ideas may seem foreign and unachievable. But deep down, under that "Walter Mitty" exterior, is a dynamic and enthusiastic individual who can't wait to get out and show the world what you can do. The key to unlocking that person lies not only in achieving your weight-loss objective but also in your willingness to embrace the fact that your success is truly the product of your own efforts.

Part of your self-image is the shell you're encased in, known as your skin. We'll cover changes in your outward appearance as it applies to that part of your body in the next chapter.

15

Skin Care following Weight-Loss Surgery

*You can know the name of a bird in all the languages
of the world, but when you're finished, you'll know
absolutely nothing whatever about the bird. . . . So let's look
at the bird and see what it's doing—that's what counts.
I learned very early the difference between knowing
the name of something and knowing something.*

—Richard Feynman, physicist

It seems that after weight-loss surgery, the thing nearly everyone becomes concerned about is an organ most people take for granted. That is the skin. This chapter is devoted to helping you understand this often overlooked organ, so uniquely affected by weight gain and loss, so you can better care for it.

The first class you take in medical school is gross anatomy. That is the study of all the body parts, big, small, and in between. The study of anatomy involves learning how all the organs, blood vessels, nerves, and bones fit together in one nice, neat package. What is often overlooked is that the package is wrapped up inside a single remarkable organ we call skin.

In addition to being the largest organ of the body, the skin is also one of the most important. We tend to take the skin for granted, perhaps because we see it and touch it every day. All the other organs, with the exception of the eyes, are hidden and are therefore quite mysterious and seemingly more important.

Recently an art exhibit came through our city called "Body Worlds." You may have seen it. The exhibition consists of a collection of anatomy dissections, some of individual organs and several entire human bodies in various poses with the skin removed. The underlying muscles, bones, and internal organs are displayed in a fascinating and artistic manner for everyone to see.

The dissection of these bodies obviously occurred after the death of the individual, and the tissues have been preserved to avoid decay. Reactions to the exhibit range from awe to disgust, because these are parts of real bodies that most people have never seen. They are always covered with ordinary old skin. By showing these dissected specimens as if performing various activities such as playing basketball or riding a horse, the artist is attempting to show what the living body would look like without its outer covering. But the fact is that human life is not possible without the protection provided by the skin.

What Is Skin and What Does It Do?

The skin is a very complex organ that provides a number of vital functions. It is both flexible and extremely tough. It is waterproof and thoroughly washable, yet requires very little in the way of maintenance. It is one of our most important sensory organs, providing us with both pleasurable touch and pain that can trigger a reflex withdrawal away from harm. It is our primary protection against bacterial invasion and provides the most important mechanism for regulating our internal temperature. It replaces itself continuously and when injured is capable of regenerating itself automatically.

It grows with us from birth to adulthood. It can stretch to meet the needs of an enlarging body, as we've all seen with obesity or pregnancy, then more or less contract back to its original size. It can be transferred from one part of the body to another, and even from one body to another and survive and grow. We can and often do neglect it and even abuse it, but it continues to serve us in all of these ways. The skin is truly one of the most amazing organs of the body.

Skin is composed of two primary layers. The top or superficial layer is called the epidermis, which is continuously replaced. The second or deep layer, the dermis, remains more or less constant.

The layer of cells that separates these two layers is called the basal layer, and it is responsible for creating the epidermis by continuously producing new cells that are progressively pushed toward the surface. As the cells get closer to the surface they tend to flatten out and die. The top of the skin is actually layers of dead cells that eventually wear away, only to be replaced by the new ones making their way toward the surface.

Melanocytes are also located within the basal layer. These are the cells that produce the skin pigment melanin. The color of the skin, which can range from extremely pale yellow to almost black, is determined both by how many melanocytes are present and how active they are at producing pigment. Exposure to ultraviolet light will temporarily stimulate these cells to produce more melanin, a process commonly known as getting a tan.

Within the skin are a number of specialized structures, each of which has an important role to play in the overall function of this organ. The one that is most obvious is the hair follicle. Hair follicles are present to one degree or another in virtually every area of the skin, and each follicle gives rise to a single hair. Generally the follicles are most numerous and arranged very close together on the top of your head, but that obviously varies from person to person. Growing out of the follicle is a shaft of hair, which is composed of very strong but dead cellular material that is held together by filaments of protein called keratin. Hair comes in a variety of colors and textures, straight or curly, and is a major contributor to our personal appearance. But that is not its job.

The main function of your hair is to improve the insulating capability of the skin. Having a lot of hair on your head can serve you very well on a cold, wintry day, and it also helps cool your scalp if you're out in the blazing sun. Each little hair follicle has a tiny little muscle attached to it called a pilo-erector muscle. When you are cold or become frightened all those tiny muscles contract, making each hair stand straight up—"a hair-raising experience." This automatic process actually serves to change the flow of air over the surface of the skin, which increases its insulating properties.

Another structure contained within the skin is the sebaceous gland. These tiny glands are intimately associated with the hair follicle. They secrete an oily substance that lubricates both the hair and the surrounding skin. People with oily skin have sebaceous glands that tend to be very active, while those with dry skin put out far less of this natural lubricant. This oily substance continuously makes its way to the surface alongside the shaft of the hair, through the tiny pores in the skin.

The skin is also the home of another type of gland, the sweat gland—not the most glamorous part of the skin, but certainly one of the most important. Sweat glands each have their own tiny pores that open to the surface. The process of sweating is a critical part of the body's temperature-regulation process. When water is secreted from these glands onto the surface of the skin, it helps cool the body through the process of evaporation: the same principle as air conditioning. On a warm day, if you were unable to sweat, your body would rapidly overheat.

Under extreme conditions the volume of water that your body can lose through this process can be as much as a liter per hour. As a band patient that is particularly important, because you may have trouble drinking enough fluids to avoid dehydration. If you become dehydrated, your body will attempt to hold on to all the water it can, and you'll eventually stop sweating. It then becomes critical to get to a cooler place and drink some water, otherwise your body temperature will start to rise uncontrollably. This life-threatening condition is known as heat stroke.

An extraordinary network of blood vessels and nerve endings is found throughout the skin. The nerve endings are particularly fascinating. It doesn't matter where the skin is touched—you feel the sensation—but it is far more sophisticated than that. You can easily tell whether you are being poked with a sharp pin or with a blunt finger. You also know the precise location of the contact. In an instant you can distinguish between the touch of a woolen scarf and a silk one. You can even feel the difference between a dry towel and one that is slightly damp. That is pretty amazing if you stop to think about it. For example, if you touch something hot, your hand will jerk back instantaneously, before you are even aware of the pain. While we take all of these things for granted, they are all possible because of the remarkable network of nerve endings contained in the skin.

Skin is affected by excess body fat but doesn't actually store the fat. Immediately beneath the skin is a layer of fatty tissue called the subcutaneous adipose tissue. That is where much of the body's stored fat is located, especially in women.

So, now that you are totally amazed by what your skin actually does for you, we need to shift back to the subject of obesity and discuss what happens to your skin as a result of weight gain and weight loss.

The Effect of Obesity on Your Skin

In most obese people the subcutaneous layer is where most of the excess fat is stored. That is especially true for obese women. As we discussed earlier, men tend to have a somewhat higher percentage of their fat stored inside the abdomen, but obese men also develop a thick layer of fat under the skin. Along with the buildup of these fatty deposits, the skin is also required to expand to accommodate the enlarging body. If the weight gain is gradual, there is a possibility that the skin can actually grow to meet the need. That is more likely in young people with healthy skin than it is in older people.

No matter the age, when weight gain is fairly rapid, or extreme, the skin may not be capable of growing fast enough, so it will merely stretch. This kind of stretching of the skin damages the dense fibrous tissues of the dermis, which provide much of the skin's strength, as well as the elastic fibers that allow the skin to rebound. In other words, the skin can be permanently damaged. The result is what we commonly call stretch marks. They are actually visual evidence of the underlying damage that has occurred as a result of weight gain.

Cellulite

The fat deposited in the subcutaneous layer isn't always smooth and uniform. Sometimes it can be quite lumpy or create dimpling of the skin. This is commonly referred to as cellulite. In reality it is simply irregular deposits of fat. It has nothing to do with the skin, except for the fact that these irregular lumps of fat cause the skin to follow their contour. The dimpling is caused by random fibrous bands that connect the skin to the deeper layers of tissue below the fat. These dense bands of tissue don't stretch as the fat accumulates, and the result is the dimpling that is sometimes called "hail damage" or "cottage cheese skin."

Treating cellulite has grown into a multimillion-dollar industry. A wide variety of lotions and creams are sold with the promise of making this "unsightly skin just disappear." Well, the fact is that cellulite is not a skin condition at all. The appearance is caused by excess fat under the skin. It may seem like the problem is improved after vigorously rubbing the area with that magic lotion, but the effect is due more to the mechanical action of messaging than any chemical that is being applied. The act of applying pressure to the skin can temporarily redistribute the underlying fat. That is why the various wraps and tight-fitting garments seem to improve cellulite as well. Liposuction has been advocated to treat cellulite, but it may actually make the problem worse because it can cause even more irregularity of the fat deposits. The best treatment for cellulite is weight loss, period.

Skin Fungus

One of the most common problems associated with obesity is the red rash that develops between the folds of skin, especially under the breasts, in the groin, and under a large overhanging abdomen. This is a fungal infection in the skin, and the medical term is intertriginous moniliasis. Everyone has tiny fungus spores on the surface of the skin, but they require certain conditions to cause an infection. You can think of skin fungus as being a close relative of the mushroom. To grow it requires a warm, moist, and dark place where food is abundant. This perfectly describes the space between the folds of skin: the deeper the fold, the more warmth, moisture, and darkness. The skin itself provides the nourishment.

Athlete's foot is caused by essentially the same fungus, and there are numerous antifungal powders and creams available to treat this condition. There are also prescription medications, both topical treatments and antifungal pills, that can help control these kinds of infections. But, unless you eliminate the environment that supports fungal growth, it will come right back. That means you need to keep the area dry and cool—not an easy task when gravity continues to slam those folds together.

Antifungal powders may help to absorb some of the moisture, but they have to be applied frequently. Placing an absorbent cloth between the layers of skin may also help, but the cloth tends to slide out and must be repositioned frequently. Probably the best treatment is to lie in a cool, dry place and expose the infected area to the light for 30 minutes to an hour, two or three times a day. It doesn't sound very practical, I know, but when combined with other antifungal treatments, it works.

This type of fungal infection frequently damages the skin, causing permanent discoloration and visible scarring. If the infection is severe enough or is present for an extended period, a secondary bacterial infection of the skin may occur. Patients with diabetes are particularly prone to both fungal and bacterial skin infections because of their impaired ability to fight infection. Fungal infections of the skin are rarely ever serious and they are almost never life threatening, but if the fungus gets into the bloodstream it can cause an extremely serious infection.

The Effect of Weight Loss on Your Skin

While gaining weight has the potential to stretch, pucker, and even injure your skin, you would assume that losing weight would undo all that. Unfortunately, that generally isn't the case. After major weight loss the excess skin can make some patients feel like a shar-pei puppy.

I get asked all the time, "How can this happen?" The answer is simple: the skin used to be full of fat; the fat went away, leaving the empty skin behind. In most cases when the skin becomes damaged by the stretching process, it loses much of its elasticity. Certainly, this varies from patient to patient and depends on many factors. The main ones are how much stretching has taken place, the part of the body involved, the duration of the obesity, the age of the patient, the general health of the skin, and how rapidly the weight is lost. You can't control most of those factors, but you can influence the health of your skin and how quickly you lose the weight.

Even damaged skin will likely retain some of its elastic properties and will tighten up with time. Losing weight slowly may allow the skin to rebound to some extent as the fat stores shrink. That is not always the case, however, especially in cases of extreme obesity. And younger patients are more likely to experience this skin retightening than older individuals, regardless of the rate of weight loss.

Fat distribution varies considerably from one person to the next. Some people carry most of their weight in and around their abdomen. Others have more fat on their hips and legs. Still others may have a very heavy chest, neck, and shoulders. As a rule, the parts of the body that are farthest from the core tend to be affected the least, so the skin of the feet and hands, the lower legs, and the forearms gets stretched less than other areas. As you lose weight the skin in these areas is much more likely to shrink back to its normal size without showing any permanent damage.

The feet and ankles can certainly become swollen, however, especially if obesity is accompanied by venous congestion and chronic swelling. In that case the problem is the accumulation of water in dependent tissues with poor circulation, called edema. All the tissues, not just the skin, become boggy as the blood pools in your feet and ankles.

The presence of chronic edema causes the skin to become thicker, and with time the color will become darker. These areas are very susceptible to ulcerations, called venous stasis ulcers, that are very slow to heal. To a lesser degree these same skin changes, especially the thickening and discoloration, can occur in any area that has become abnormally dependent. It's common on the underside of the breast, the inner thighs, and especially the bottom of a large abdominal "apron," called a pannus.

Because the skin of the upper arms and thighs is subject to more stretching, it tends to remain that way even after significant weight loss. The folds of skin in the groin area are also more likely to have suffered from fungal infection because of moisture and irritation. Even with major weight loss these folds and the infections that occur there are likely to persist. The same thing can be said about virtually every other area that has been subjected to chronic obesity.

Peter's Story

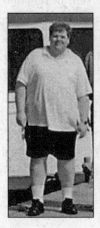
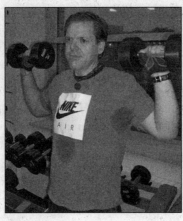

(Left) Peter, pre-op, 407.2 pounds.

(Right) Peter, three years post-op, 219 pounds.

My sister and brother-in-law are both physicians, and they were both concerned along with the rest of my family about my weight. So Christmas of 2001, my brother-in-law, whose specialty is internal medicine, trapped me in the car for over an hour. He took advantage of the opportunity to lecture me about my weight and weight-loss surgery. He knew I'd done the various weight-loss diets and even some weight-loss drugs. I did well on a couple, losing 80 to 90 pounds, but the pounds came back, along with friends.

I told him I'd think about it, and I did for an entire year. I looked at the various surgical options available and decided it was the band I was interested in. In March of 2003 I made the appointment with my band surgeon. I went twice, and he answered all of my questions each time. I booked the surgery for June of 2003, but it got canceled because of the SARS crisis in Canada, where I live.

Pre-op I weighed in at 407.2 pounds, and I'm 6 feet, 1 inch, so my BMI was 52. My condition had the depressing title "super obese." I chose to get the Swedish 9cc band. I've had no complications. Actually, that's just blown my mind. I haven't vomited, and I've had no reflux. I did have reflux before the band. Basically, the band is keeping the acid from rising up past it, so it cured my acid reflux.

The only problem I've had was an incident with French bread. I'd finished one scrambled egg and a slice of French bread when intense pain started in my chest where the band is. So I went to the sink, thinking I'd throw up. I didn't; I had to wait it out. But I haven't had a slice of bread since. I now avoid any bread that balls up if I roll it between my fingertips. Once in a blue moon I do have sliming, but never followed by vomiting. That's happened when I've rushed eating. So essentially I feel I've had no problems at all.

The very first week after surgery I lost 17 pounds. I thought it was water weight. The following week I took off another 6 pounds. It kept going like that and I lost 205 pounds altogether in 14 months, which averages out to about 4 pounds a week. I remember that once or twice I lost only 1 or 2 pounds one week and got annoyed.

Now, three years post-op, I couldn't be more happy. I've kept the weight off. I'm 219 now. I'd like to be at 215, and my lowest weight was 202. But at 202 some people said that I looked too thin, that my face looked emaciated, and I remember my port was sticking out. I had a sternal placement of my port, and it looked like I'd swallowed a golf ball. So I asked my band surgeon to move it during one of my plastic surgeries; it's now an inch away from my belly button and doesn't stick out.

All my fills have been done under fluoroscopy. For some reason my surgeon cannot do them the other way. I have 5ccs in my 9cc band now, and I'm delighted with that. My surgeon did remove some of my fill for the first of my plastic surgeries, but he's recently told me that there's no need for that anymore for surgery not related to the band.

Normally exercise is a big part of my weight loss. I work out three times a week at the gym, since I live near one. I do upper and lower body work for an hour and a half. I swim twice a week for more than an hour. I take a brisk walk for an hour a day, and in the summer I extend that to two or three hours. Most people say walking doesn't do much, but I enjoy it. I also participate not so consistently in other activities, such as yoga, pilates, and squash.

My life is very different now. This is a guy who never used to exercise before the band. I was very lazy. Now I really do enjoy all types of exercise. I'm not demoralized by being out of breath all the time, as I was doing ordinary activities. I enjoy being able to blend into the crowd, not standing out, not having people stare at me.

My pants went from a size 54 to a size 36. My shirts went from a 4x or 5x down to Large. I feel so much better about myself. I didn't mind any longer looking at my reflection in store windows. Now I actually go out of my way to look.

I enjoy the non-scale victory things, too, like no longer needing a seatbelt extender on the plane. I used to ask for the extender in a sneaky way, whisper to attendant, and she'd bring it to me discreetly. The last flight, I had slack in my seatbelt and I could pull down the tray table. Before, my meals used to slide off the tray table because I was too big for it to lie flat.

I enjoy not having to go to the big and tall shop. I now buy designer stuff at discount prices. Though, there for a while, I spent too much money on clothes. When I was at 400 pounds, I bought what I had to. I never threw anything away, so I kept all my clothes from the way up. I recently got rid of 10 garbage bags full of clothes. I did keep one pair of the fat pants, and now both my legs fit in one leg of those pants. I have a photo of me with another band patient. She is in one leg of the pants and I am in the other.

Other medical problems cleared up besides the acid reflux. I had sleep apnea and needed a CPAP machine. Once I'd lost 100 pounds, that went away. And I had severe knee pain, and that's gone.

I think my most important piece of advice for other band people is to follow the rules most of the time. I never drink beverages with meals, and I wait an hour afterward to drink anything. I don't have pop at all; no beer, either. I eat protein first, then vegetables, then carbs. I do have cookies once in a while. I used to have a whole bag at a sitting, but now I have two or three and stop. I'd also caution people not to eat so they throw up regularly.

I think the band is a great tool, and everyone should know about it. My background is in science, and the idea in science is to look for the simplest theory or approach to solve a problem. I think the band fits that description—it's a terrific and simple solution.

Minimizing the Damage

We all want young, healthy skin, right? Unfortunately, as you get older your skin ages along with you, and there is no such thing as a fountain of youth. Time marches on for all of us. But some people have skin that is more youthful in appearance. For some, this is genetic; they're blessed with naturally healthy skin. For others, their skin remains healthy because they work at it. They avoid using harsh soaps, apply moisturizing lotions regularly, and perhaps most important, they stay out of the sun.

Did you ever wonder why your skin tans as a result of being out in the sun? As I mentioned earlier in this chapter, ultraviolet rays stimulate melanocytes to make more melanin pigment—that's "how" the skin tans. But the reason the skin gets darker is that the melanin helps block those ultraviolet rays from penetrating into the deeper layer of the skin, the dermis. That is where real damage can occur to the blood vessels, nerves, and supporting structures. The pigment is the body's way of trying to protect itself from the harmful UV rays.

With prolonged exposure to the sun or other artificial sources of ultraviolet light (tanning beds), the result will eventually be permanent damage to your skin. Over time your skin will become leathery, thicker, and less flexible than normal. You'll also have more wrinkles, and you may even lose some of your sensitivity to touch. When chronic sun damage is combined with major weight loss, it can create some very unsightly results.

Ultraviolet radiation also increases your risk of developing skin cancer, including one of the more aggressive forms of malignancy, melanoma. That may not have anything to do with obesity and weight loss, but it is an important message to take into account when caring for your skin. The bottom line: for healthier skin, stay out of the sun and the tanning bed. If you are going to be out in the sun, you should either wear protective clothing or apply a sunscreen with an SPF (Sun Protection Factor) rating of at least 15 to all exposed areas.

Skin-care Products

If you go to any drug store, department store, hair salon, or grocery store, you can't help but be exposed to the unbelievable number of skin-care products that are on the market. If you go online, the selection is seemingly limitless, and the cost of some of these products is utterly astounding. It is well beyond the scope of this book for me even to attempt to comment on the relative effectiveness of any specific lotion, cream, ointment, salve, liniment, gel, body rub, or balm.

Without question, many skin-care products can help promote healthy skin, either by promoting healing or providing protection. The lubricating and protective effects of natural substances like lanolin, an oil secreted by the sebaceous gland of certain sheep, have been recognized for centuries. Interestingly, lanolin is one of the main ingredients in shoe polish because of its ability to help keep "tanned leather" soft.

There are many "natural" products such as aloe vera, camellia oil, cocoa butter, coconut oil, lavender oil, avocados, seaweed, emu oil, green tea, etc., etc., etc., that are touted as being capable of rejuvenating, regenerating, tightening, firming, or (my favorite) "youthening" the skin, whatever that means. There are even some skin-care products that say they offer breast enhancement! But it's important to recognize that manufacturers of skin-care products don't have to demonstrate the effectiveness of their products the way drug manufacturers do. Skin-care products are classified as cosmetics, and therefore they are not regulated by the Food and Drug Administration (FDA). The following statement comes directly from the FDA website, and it sums up this issue pretty well: "The Food, Drug, and Cosmetic Act defines drugs as those products that cure, treat, mitigate or prevent disease or that affect the structure or function of the human body. While drugs are subject to an intensive review and approval process by FDA, cosmetics are not approved by FDA prior to sale. If a product has drug properties, it must be approved as a drug."

For those patients who are experiencing problems with their skin, the best advice is to consult a dermatologist—a physician who specializes in the diagnosis and treatment of skin conditions. In the long run, getting the advice of a dermatologist may save you a small fortune in over-the-counter treatments. But even the dermatologist isn't going to have an answer for all that excess skin that's hanging off your now more slender body. For that, you'll likely need a nip and a tuck, which is the subject of the next chapter.

16

Plastic Surgery
following Weight Loss

*We all have big changes in our lives
that are more or less a second chance.*

—Harrison Ford, actor,
from *Harrison Ford: Imperfect Hero* by Garry Jenkins

After all your hard work, you've finally reached your goal weight. Or perhaps you've reached a final plateau that is close enough to what you wanted, and now you're left with a bunch of extra skin. In the last chapter, we looked in detail at skin and how it's affected by weight gain and weight loss.

Now that you've lost weight, and your skin isn't what you'd like it to be, you're probably asking yourself, "Should I have plastic surgery?" For many patients the answer frequently goes something like this: "Well, I've come this far, I might as well go all the way." Others are more reluctant, either because of cost or risk. Depending on how noticeable that extra skin is, you may not want to bother. With time there may be some additional shrinkage, but it is very difficult to know to what degree. This chapter is intended to "tie everything up"—pun clearly intended.

If you are considering plastic surgery, it is important that you know all the facts. What is possible? What isn't possible? What exactly does plastic surgery entail? When is a good time to have it? What are the risks? Who should you go to? Let's start with the last question first.

Choosing a Plastic Surgeon

We usually think of the word "plastic" as referring to a synthetic material that is chemically produced specifically to replace a natural material like wood or iron. But in surgery the word "plastic" is an adjective defined in Taber's Cyclopedic Medical Dictionary as "capable of being molded." And "plastic surgery" is defined as "surgery for the restoration, repair, or reconstruction of body structures."

A plastic surgeon is a doctor who has completed additional training specifically in the performance of these procedures. He or she is a specialist in the field. However, not all plastic surgeons routinely perform recontouring procedures specifically for patients following major weight loss. So, in addition to finding a surgeon who is certified by the American Board of Plastic Surgery, you should also inquire about specific experience in the area of body contouring following weight loss.

It is common for patients to choose a plastic surgeon based on the recommendation of a friend who has had one or more procedures by that particular surgeon. You can also ask your primary doctor or the surgeon who performed your band operation whom they would recommend. Having someone you trust make a recommendation can add significantly to your confidence, even before you meet the surgeon. But, ultimately, the decision about which doctor you have do your surgery should be totally up to you, and based on your own assessment.

When you go in for an initial consultation with a plastic surgeon, the first thing you should find out is how much experience the surgeon has with body contouring after weight loss. There are many very talented plastic surgeons who have great reputations for doing various cosmetic operations but who may not be familiar with the special circumstances surrounding your particular situation. What you should be looking for is someone who takes a special interest in this area. That doesn't necessarily mean that's all they do, but your results are likely to be better with someone who has some experience.

Don't just dive into all the things you want done. Take some time to get acquainted and see if this is someone you can relate to and who seems genuinely to care about you. The surgeon will want to understand your entire medical history, not just your weight loss, and he or she will want to take a careful look at you before making any recommendations.

You probably won't have to ask them to show you photographs. Most plastic surgeons have numerous before and after photos of patients whom they have operated on. Make sure they are showing you their results, not those out of a textbook or some other surgeon's experience. Also, realize that it is only natural for the surgeon to show you his or her best work, so you can anticipate seeing some really spectacular results. Not every patient ends up with spectacular results. Ask to see pictures of what the surgeon considers average results, and even some poor results. You need to be prepared for all the possibilities.

If there was ever a time for a second opinion, this is it. Many plastic surgeons offer free initial evaluations, but even if you have to pay for two or three consultations, it will be worth it if they ultimately help you make the right choice. Remember, this is like hiring someone to design and remodel your home. Take your time and get a few bids. If at all possible, get some references and telephone them. Understand that the surgeon is likely to give you only the names of patients who are very satisfied with their results. Even so, you can get some very useful insights into what you can expect by asking questions about the doctor's attention to detail, as well as the attitude and responsiveness of the staff.

Checklist: Looking for a Plastic Surgeon

- ✓ Ask doctors you know for referrals.
- ✓ Ask for referrals from other patients.
- ✓ Get two or three surgeons to talk to.
- ✓ Take your time and get a few bids. This is like remodeling your house. You want to feel knowledgeable and comfortable with the surgeon you choose.
- ✓ Does the surgeon care about you and your medical history?
- ✓ Do you get the feeling that they have your interests at heart? Are they in a hurry for you to get started? (That is not a good sign.)
- ✓ Does the surgeon have experience with body contouring after weight loss?
- ✓ Ask to see before and after photos, not only of great outcomes but also of average and poor outcomes. You need to be prepared for all the possibilities.
- ✓ Are there patients you can talk to?
- ✓ What is the doctor's attitude and responsiveness, as well as the responsiveness of the staff?

When Should I Start Plastic Surgery?

Speaking of time, the timing of any plastic surgery can be critical, so make sure that you and the surgeon agree on an appropriate time to begin the makeover process. I have had some patients who were extremely impatient and wanted to have something done long before they had finished losing weight. Most of the time taking that approach ends up being wasteful and creates less than satisfactory results.

It's generally a good idea to wait six months to a year after you have achieved your maximum weight loss (meaning you've stopped losing weight for that long) before having plastic surgery. Any sooner and you run the risk that you may lose more weight, which might require another operation to trim away additional excess skin. You also want to make sure that your weight is stable, since some people regain some of the weight they have lost within the first year. You could be all neatly repackaged only to start the stretching process over again. And scar tissue doesn't stretch as well as the initial skin did.

Be Prepared for Scars

It is important to recognize that there will be scars. There is no such thing as scar-free surgery. Essentially, what you are doing with plastic surgery is trading extra skin for scars. Now, some procedures have fewer noticeable scars than other, and some surgeons seem to have better outcomes than others, but they will all tell you that it is not possible to predict exactly what your scars will look like once the incisions have healed.

As a rule, body contouring requires the removal of huge pieces of skin, and therefore long scars. In some cases these can be partially hidden, but you will always be able to see them. Be fully prepared for what they are likely to look like before you go ahead.

What to Lift and What to Leave

Some patients want only limited changes, such as a partial face lift or removal of their excess upper-arm skin. Others may want multiple areas lifted and others enhanced. It is critical that you talk candidly with the surgeon about what you would like. There is nothing wrong with creating a list of what you consider "must do's," "might do's," and "wish I could do's."

Don't be shy to list everything you can think of; it doesn't mean you are going to do any of it at this point. It will give the surgeon a clear understanding of what your priorities are, so he or she can develop a plan that meets your needs as efficiently as possible. You may even discover that one or more of the procedures on your wish list are easier to get than you thought.

Once you have decided on precisely what you want, you and the surgeon will need to agree on the timing and sequencing, if multiple procedures are involved. You may want to have several different procedures performed at the same time, either to save money or because you're in a hurry, or both. And some procedures are more easily combined than others.

A prudent plastic surgeon will not recommend initiating your plastic surgery plan until your weight has been stable for at least six months. He or she will also recommend which procedures you can safely combine along with an appropriate interval between procedures, often several months. This is necessary to give you time to recover from the stress of the operation and heal the incisions. Just remember that these procedures are much like your original bariatric surgery, totally elective. Make sure that both you and your surgeon are comfortable with the strategy before you go with it.

The Procedures

Body contouring involves more than just lopping off some hanging skin and sewing you back up. The process takes on somewhat of an artistic air, with you as the lump of clay and the plastic surgeon as the sculptor. The objective is to reshape your skin to match the original appearance as closely as possible.

Some parts are easier than others, but it is possible to modify virtually every part. Doing so can also result in the loss of several more pounds, but don't confuse this side benefit of plastic surgery with your overall weight-loss program. It's simply a bonus, not a substitute for diet and exercise.

Face and Neck

Some of the most dramatic results are obtained by lifting the sagging skin of the face and neck. These are areas that are always visible, so eliminating those jowls, the gobbler neck, or the bags under your eyes can make you look years younger. These procedures can also be done with very little visible scarring, since the incisions can usually be hidden in the hairline or behind the line of the jaw. Not all facelifts are they same. Be sure that you and the surgeon have agreed on what will and what won't be lifted. You may or may not need a complete makeover.

There is a procedure called a "thread lift" that has been widely publicized as an inexpensive and quick alternative to a formal facelift. It involves using a series of sutures that are threaded through the skin and are then secured to other tissues higher up in the face to suspend the sagging skin with very minimal incisions. In theory it sounds good, but it is usually only recommended for young people looking for a minor lift. The results can be somewhat unpredictable, and the lift it provides typically doesn't last as long as a more traditional facelift.

Arms

One of the more noticeable and annoying excess skin problems, especially for women who lose a large amount of weight, is the upper arm area. The appearance is commonly called "bat wings" because when the arms are extended straight out, the skin droops down dramatically from the elbows back toward the chest. For many women this is the first thing they have addressed with plastic surgery, because the problem is obvious when they wear anything that is short sleeve or sleeveless. You have just lost a bunch of weight and are buying new clothes that you want to flatter that new body, only to have these "bat wings" visible as a reminder of your recent past. There is really no way to hide them other than long sleeves, and even then the excess skin takes up considerable space inside the garment, making it feel too tight in the arms.

Addressing the upper arm skin is not as technically difficult as some of the other areas of the body, but it does leave visible scars down the arms. There are some surgeons who claim to get good results by pulling all the skin up into the arm pit and thus hiding the scar, and that may be possible if the problem is relatively minor to start with. When large amounts of skin need to be removed, it probably won't work nearly as well as an incision down the length of the upper arm.

Most patients are thrilled with their new, slimmer arms and don't seem to mind the scars, but be sure to look closely at the pictures you are shown before having this procedure. Make sure that you are comfortable with the location and extent of the scars, because you will see them every day for the rest of your life.

Janet's Story

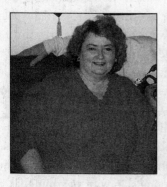 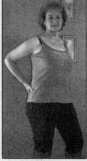

(Left) Janet, pre-op, over 300 pounds.

(Right) Janet, three years post-op, about 170 pounds.

I think my starting weight was 289 when I first saw Dr. Sewell, and I'm 5 feet, 6 inches. I'd lost about 30 pounds on my own, so my top weight was well over 300 pounds. I'd tried everything else, and all of the diets worked to a point. I'm not saying that they're bad for anyone else. Everyone is dif-

ferent, and different things work for other people. But while people can argue that obesity is a head thing all they want, I was always hungry. I'd try
starving myself and I'd get nauseated. And I didn't make good choices
when I chose food.

When I started researching band surgery all I heard about was gastric
bypass, and I thought there was no way I'd allow my insides to be
rerouted. I went to another doctor's seminar and heard about the band. I
was married at the time and my husband was leery, so I let it drop. Later,
when I was getting divorced, I e-mailed my ex, said this is what I want to
do, and this is what I need from you to do it. He agreed to help.

Dr. Sewell put my band in on April 2, 2003, and by early June I'd lost 40
pounds. I've lost about 120 pounds altogether in the four years I've had
the band.

I've always been extremely active. I used to shock people, because
people would be surprised what I did. I hiked and did a lot of things. Even
so, I notice a difference in my energy now that I have more of it and I feel
better.

The second biggest thing I noticed was the change in people's attitudes. I was always friendly and outgoing, but a lot of people seemed to
think that I suddenly got a brain. My opinions seem more valuable, and it
really kind of irritated me because it's so unfair. But I notice now that instead of having to pretend to be confident and assured, I am confident
and assured. The weight loss gave me a freedom. I feel good about what
I'm doing, and I feel good about my life. It's not a compelling feeling anymore that I have to make them feel good and I have to make them understand what I'm doing. Now I can let them not understand. I still go into a
store to buy clothes and I walk to the women's department first instead of
the misses. I have to correct myself. I was in 26/28, and now I'm in a
10/12. I have some stretchy jeans that are 8/10 and some jeans that are
14, so a lot depends on the brand.

I'm a nurse, and I work two jobs because my parents are in assisted living I need the income. I do phone triage for a hospital. When I applied for
the second job at the high school, I realized I probably wouldn't have gotten the job before because of my weight. But not only did I get the job but
I'm also taking a trip to Europe this summer with the foreign language club
at the school. We're going to Spain, Germany, and France, and we'll be
gone for two weeks. I feel comfortable doing this trip knowing that I'll not
have to wedge into a little, narrow seat in the plane.

In fact, I'm more comfortable everywhere. I go into a movie theater and
sit down and don't have to worry about wedging people out beside me. I
can bend straight over to tie my shoes. I can bend over and reach something under a piece of furniture, instead of getting down on the floor and
crawling over to pick something up. All those little things mean more to me
than anything. It's still amazing to me.

My band slipped once, and I had to have it redone. I knew something
was wrong because I had such bad reflux. I'd always had some reflux, but

this was very tough. I didn't go to Dr. Sewell, though, because I didn't feel it was that important. Then I ate a small salad and it went down, but I kept burping a lot. The burping was nauseating, and it was foul tasting. I was getting sick to my stomach, and I threw up rotted lettuce two days later. And that's when I felt I needed to get it checked out. It was so foul tasting that I was still gagging when I went to see Dr. Sewell, and the smell was still in my nose. He did the upper GI and saw that the band had slipped.

The repair was easy, and I was in the hospital a day. I scheduled it so I had several days off. When I first woke up I started taking fluids again. I thought, "This stuff is going down easy." The most I've ever carried in my band is 1.5ccs. But this time, when it was time for a fill, I had him put only 0.5cc in it. And that has been just enough to keep me honest. If I try to eat too much the band is like a fist grabbing me and going, "No you don't." I wish they'd had this 30 years ago. But on the other hand, I wouldn't try to talk anyone else into it. To be honest, it's a good and bad thing. You have to be ready to do this or you won't be successful.

I have an overweight friend whose husband is encouraging her to get a band. But I told her I wouldn't try to talk her into it. She was shocked and asked why. I said that all you ever talk about are the potential problems and how much you'll miss the food you love. That tells me you're not ready.

There are times, I'd give my eye teeth to have a huge steak and baked potato. Steak now is out of the question. No matter how much I chew it, it's like it gets bigger in my mouth. And beef is very heavy on my stomach. But would I have the weight back so I could enjoy those foods again? No way. Food used to be extremely important to me. You don't totally lose that when you've been there so long, but it doesn't take much thought for me to make the choice I want, and that's to be smaller.

Some people don't seem to care, and find ways to eat around the band. Those people are not going to succeed. Someone else I know got a band, and they told me they didn't want to exercise and never intended to exercise. They said they'd paid enough for the band that they didn't feel they should have to do anything more. I answered that if I'd known they felt that way, I would have suggested they think about doing something besides a band.

I think some people I know are internally really angry with me for losing weight. One of my overweight friends said to me that when I talk about the band it irritates her and that it "makes me just hate you." It isn't like I talk about the band all the time. I wait until someone asks me before I comment. I've heard that when you're overweight you lose friends because you're overweight. When you lose the weight and get thin, you find out which of your friends are real friends, because the ones who leave never were.

I've had two plastic surgeries. My primary care physician said I'm too old to be doing all this plastic surgery. But I had my arms done, and at the same time the plastic surgeon did a lateral chest incision halfway under each breast to give me a mini lift. I don't want breast implants. The latest I had took skin from all the way around me at the waist and gave me a tummy tuck along with a butt and thigh lift. On the plastic surgery, I was determined to make sure I did it right. I feel like I've had good results, but someone younger would have better results because they're younger. I lost weight with each surgery, but I lost 13 to 15 pounds with surgery around my waist alone.

My grown son has been transferred back with his job, so he lives near me, and now I have six grandchildren nearby. And I can keep up with those grandchildren. With the weight loss, so many good things have happened, I wonder when it'll stop. I'm extremely thankful. I believe it was divine intervention.

Breasts

This is probably the most subjective of all areas of body contouring. What exactly is a normal breast? Following weight loss, most women find their breasts sagging. That is because the average breast is composed of more than 50 percent fat, and in obese women that number may be closer to 90 percent. So when you lose a lot of weight, the breast is one of those places where it shows the most.

To address the problem of sagging breasts isn't just a matter of removing skin. Any breast lift by necessity must also include the repositioning of the nipple-areola, so that the breast looks normal. This usually requires a "keyhole" shaped incision with removal of the excess skin from the bottom of the breast: the nipple area is moved up, and the skin closed beneath it. This creates a scar that goes completely around the areola (the dark skin around he nipple) and then extends straight down to the bottom of the breast and then under the entire breast. Because the scars are on the bottom of the breast, they are not generally visible even in a low-cut blouse, but typically they will be quite obvious to you every time you shower.

Depending on how much of your breast tissue has disappeared with weight loss, some women actually have their breasts enhanced with implants. This can be done at the same time as the lift and may greatly improve the overall appearance. But again, this is an extremely subjective issue, and you should do what feels right to you.

Men who lose a large amount of weight may also be plagued with sagging skin on their chest and around their breasts. The same type of procedure can be performed with only minor modifications to help create a more chiseled male figure.

Abdomen and Trunk

Most obese people carry much of their weight in and around their waistline. This often leads to a large, protuberant abdomen that hangs over the beltline, called an abdominal pannus, or "apron." Even without weight loss, some people opt to have this large fatty apron surgically removed with a procedure called a panniculectomy. That is most often done to help heal the skin under the pannus, or in conjunction with other internal abdominal operations simply to get it out of the way. The procedure doesn't usually lead to the kind of cosmetic result most patients are looking for after weight-loss surgery.

The "tummy tuck," otherwise known as an abdominoplasty, is the operation most commonly performed to get rid of that excess skin on the abdomen. I often chuckle when patients ask why I won't do just a little tummy tuck for them "while I'm in there." First, I don't do that procedure, and second, there's no such thing as a little tummy tuck. This is usually a major undertaking that may take several hours.

This procedure recontours the entire abdomen by removing the skin of the pannus, repositioning the belly button (umbilicus) back up to the middle of the abdomen, and sometimes even involves tightening the abdominal muscles. The scars can generally be hidden well below the waistline, but there will be a circular scar around the belly button.

If the front of your abdomen is the only concern, a standard abdominoplasty may be all you need. However, if your skin is sagging all the way around your torso, it may not be enough. The entire trunk area can be addressed with a procedure that extends all the way around, called a circumferential body lift or belt lipectomy. You can think of it as an extended tummy tuck that removes excess skin from your flanks and back and even lifts the skin of the buttocks and the outer aspects of the thighs. This is a big operation and should probably not be combined with other procedures.

Legs

The body lift may address the outer part of the upper thighs, but it doesn't do anything for all that extra skin hanging from the inner thigh. The approach to this area is much like that for the upper arm, and not uncommonly plastic surgeons will recommend they be addressed at the same time. The incisions and ultimately the scars will extend down the inner thigh from the groin area to near the knee. One of the most pleasant results of this operation can be simply that your thighs don't rub together all the time, eliminating the constant chafing of your skin in that sensitive area.

Minimizing the Scars

For patients who have lost a lot of weight, these plastic procedures are a trade-off—excess skin for permanent scars. No matter what you may have heard or want to believe, scars don't go away. But some are very obvious, while others are hardly noticeable. What is it that makes the difference? There is no quick answer to this question because the appearance of each individual scar depends on a number of factors. Some are controllable and some are not.

If the scar looks great, it is tempting to give the surgeon all the credit, and certainly his or her skill and experience play an important role. But scar tissue is part of your body's healing response to any injury. Some people naturally create dense, thick scars, yet others seem to heal with minimal visible scars. The same surgeon, performing the same procedure on two different patients, may be hailed as a hero by one, while the other may think the surgeon must have done something wrong based solely on the appearance of the scars.

There are some important things that the surgeon can do to minimize scarring, and they have to do with the direction of the incisions, the type and number of sutures used, the physical manipulation of the tissues, and perhaps most important, minimizing tension on the healing incision. Rest assured that all of these things and a whole lot more are part of every plastic surgeon's training.

The issue of tension is one that deserves some additional discussion simply because it is so important, and it is something that you can help control. Whenever two edges of the skin are sewn together, the ideal situation is for them to come together easily without any stress or tension. But if there is a gap between the two edges the skin will need to be stretched to some degree to allow the two edges to join. This creates some tension on the skin, which tries to pull the incision apart while the healing process is trying to knit the two edges together. The result is usually a wider, more obvious scar.

Surgeons will do everything possible to minimize this tension by mobilizing the edges of the skin so they will come together easily. But after the operation, any swelling under the incision will tend to stretch the skin and contribute to tension on the suture line. That is where you can actually help yourself.

Following your operation the plastic surgeon will likely recommend that you wear either an elastic bandage or some type of tight-fitting garment for a period of time. He or she may also suggest that ice packs or cold compresses be applied to certain areas periodically for a few days after surgery. Both of these recommendations are made specifically to reduce swelling in the operative site. In doing so, you will not only reduce the amount of pain you experience but also help to prevent swelling and tension across the healing skin—and the result will be a better scar.

You'll recall that in the last chapter we talked some about various skin-care products and what they can and can't do. This subject invariably comes up whenever the discussion turns to surgical scars. "Isn't there something I can put on this scar to make it go away?" Again, scars never go away, but what they look like can be influenced to a degree by how you treat them. The use of pressure applied directly to healing skin by either a tight bandage or elastic garment has been demonstrated to help decrease the extent of scarring. In patients recovering from major burns, the use of custom-fitted masks, gloves, and sleeves for several months can dramatically improve the appearance and flexibility of even the most horrific scars. Extreme measures like that are typically neither necessary nor practical following most routine plastic surgery procedures. However, as I mentioned earlier, some surgeons will suggest that you wear a tight-fitting garment for a period of time to help reduce the amount of scarring you experience.

Various ointments containing vitamin E or silicone or other substances may help to keep the developing scar tissue soft and pliable. Many surgeons believe that it helps, so they often recommend that it be applied two or three times a day. Some even advocate that you buy vitamin E capsules and break them open to apply the concentrated liquid vitamin directly to the scar. No one really knows what vitamin E does to the skin or to the development of scar tissue. From a purely scientific standpoint there is no proof that this complex molecule, which is only partially absorbed by the skin, has any influence on healing whatsoever. Nevertheless, some people swear by it, and it probably doesn't do any harm unless you apply it too soon after your surgery. However, to be perfectly clear, you should never put anything on your incision sites without first getting the okay from your surgeon.

Liposuction

The same patients who ask about the tummy tuck "while you're in there" often suggest, "Why don't you just suck out some of that excess fat while you're there?" There isn't a surgeon alive who hasn't heard that at least once. Perhaps that message was what gave rise to the whole idea of liposuction, or maybe the patients got the idea because they had heard about the procedure. Either way, it is certainly possible to suck out some of the fatty tissue from under the skin using long metal tubes inserted through tiny skin incisions. This process is called liposuction, and it is not a weight-loss procedure!

Plastic surgeons sometimes use liposuction to supplement body contouring, but the process does not remove any of the excess skin. It can remove minor irregular bulges of fat in small areas, and is generally used as a "touch up" procedure after the major skin-removal operation has completely healed. Sometimes liposuction is combined with minor scar revisions as the "artist's finishing touches." Liposuction can cause significant bleeding under the skin with major bruising, which is usually only temporary. Even so, wearing a pressure dressing or elastic garment is generally a good idea following this kind of procedure.

Surgical Risks

Some plastic surgery procedures can be done under local anesthesia in the doctor's office, but that is not usually the case with body contouring. The extent of the incisions and the length of the procedures usually require general anesthesia. Likewise, because of the potential for bleeding during major procedures, some surgeons recommend having blood available for transfusion. This can even be your own blood that you donated a few weeks in advance. For these reasons, as well as others, most of these procedures are performed in a hospital or short-stay surgical facility, rather than the doctor's office. And, having the support services of a hospital can make it much easier to deal with any unforeseen problems.

After losing all that weight, patients tend to be healthier than they were going into the band surgery. The result is that nearly every surgical risk has been reduced. Underlying illnesses such as diabetes and high blood pressure may have improved, but it's important to realize that all of the potential surgical risks discussed earlier in the book still exist. They include possible problems with anesthesia, blood clots, heart problems, pneumonia, and so on.

Don't assume that just because you've had surgery before without a hitch you are bullet proof. Surgery is a bit like flying an airplane. It is an unnatural act that goes very smoothly most of the time. When something goes wrong it may be due to outside influences beyond anyone's control, but bad situations are far less likely if you follow a standardized "preflight check list." Be sure to discuss all the potential risks with your surgeon, and then do everything "by the book."

Avoiding infection is something that every surgeon strives for because infections can delay healing, increase scarring, and even risk the life of the patient. Fortunately, body contouring procedures are associated with a relatively low rate of infection, generally in the 1 to 2 percent range. Preoperative and postoperative antibiotics are routinely used, and along with careful skin preparation they help keep this risk to a minimum. Patients with diabetes or poor circulation are at higher risk for infection, as are those who have a history of staph infections.

The skin generally has great blood supply, and even when a large flap of skin is lifted away from the underlying tissues, it can survive based on the network of tiny blood vessels in the dermis. But in patients with diabetes, and particularly in patients who smoke, the blood supply of the skin may be severely compromised. The edges of the skin flaps may not get enough blood and oxygen to stay alive. If any part of the skin dies, it will need to be removed, creating a major defect. This will lead to increased scarring and may require more surgery, including possibly even skin grafts. If you stop smoking, even for just a few weeks, you can help reduce this risk, and breathing supplemental oxygen for a time after surgery may also be of some benefit. Some plastic surgeons will not perform procedures on smokers. It would be a good idea to stop smoking permanently anyway, so perhaps this will give you the incentive.

Recovery

Following a laparoscopic AGB operation, most people take only a week or so to recover. Plastic surgery is not laparoscopic surgery. The recovery is typically more prolonged, and depends in large part on what procedure is done. After a minor face or neck lift you may be fully functional within just a few days, but it can take six to eight weeks to bounce back from a circumferential body lift.

To a large extent your recovery time will also depend on what kind of work you do, how physically demanding it is, and your general health. Talk to your surgeon about this in advance so that you can make the necessary preparations. I have heard more than one patient complain after the fact about their struggles trying to go back to work after a body sculpting procedure when they hadn't allowed enough time to be fully ready.

It is important to get back into your exercise routine as soon as you are able. Don't use this as an excuse to take several months off; you may not ever get back into it, and you sure don't want to start gaining your weight back. Your surgeon should be able to give you a good idea of what sorts of exercises you can do and when you can begin.

Medical Necessity and Insurance

No discussion of plastic surgery would be complete without at least mentioning insurance. As a rule, most heath insurance companies are not going to cover elective recontouring of your body, no matter how much you argue with them. Your policy almost certainly has language in it that specifically excludes cosmetic surgery.

However, it may be possible to get some procedures covered by insurance if you can show they are medically necessary. This doesn't mean that you're going to get anywhere just because your doctor is willing to write a letter stating the importance of skin removal. It can be pretty hard to prove that chafing under your arms or between your thighs constitutes a medical condition requiring an operation that costs several thousand dollars.

The removal of the abdominal pannus or other areas of excess skin may be approved by some insurance carriers as necessary to treat a major fungal skin infection. But they are likely to require several opinions to that effect from doctors other than the surgeon who is treating you. A breast lift can also be considered as part of a breast reduction procedure, and these operations are sometimes covered by insurance. It usually requires you to show that the weight of the breast is causing neck, shoulder, or back pain. Again, this can be an uphill climb if you've just lost 75 or 100 pounds.

Certainly you should make every reasonable effort to get the benefits you are entitled to, and your plastic surgeon's staff will undoubtedly be able to help guide you through the process. They may even have some tips that you haven't thought of. If you're truthful and accurate in your arguments, who knows? All your insurance company can do is say no—or maybe yes!

Conclusion

The most important message I can offer, and the reason this book was written, is to encourage you to do what you believe is right for you. Don't let someone else discourage you based on their bias. Don't fall victim to your own self-defeated attitude that tries to convince you that you can't change your life for the better. Don't even let your doctor's reluctance to recommend weight-loss surgery dictate what medical conditions you must endure.

And finally, don't let an insurance company's denial stand in the way of achieving your success, whether it is getting plastic surgery near the end of your journey or getting an AGB to begin the process. Listen to your own heart, and find a way. It may be the greatest thing you will ever do for yourself.

17

Living with Someone Who Has an AGB

Great services are not canceled
by one act or by one single error.
—Benjamin Disraeli

Beginning in the 1970s and maybe even the decade earlier, Americans as a whole seemed to shift toward a more self-indulgent, self-absorbed, "me first" way of thinking. Subsequently, our entire culture has followed that trend. The measure of an individual's worth has become more about what they have than who they are and what they do for others. So, what does this have to do with bariatric surgery? The answer is—everything.

The obesity epidemic is in many respects the direct result of our cultural shift toward self-gratification and our prosperity as a nation. Self-indulgence has not only become acceptable, it is encouraged: witness the "super-size me" phenomenon. When an individual comes to the realization they need help with their obesity and chooses bariatric surgery, they are actually bucking the system. The surrounding culture doesn't change. The patient may be personally committed to making major lifestyle changes, but all of the outside influences that helped promote their obesity are still active. This may even include the opinions and behaviors of the people who are closest to them.

Perhaps the most important determining factor in the success of any AGB patient beyond their own personal commitment is the understanding and support of those with whom they live and work every day. Without a support system, the pressures of day-to-day living within an environment that hasn't changed will frequently lead to failure. This places a pretty heavy burden on spouses, family members, and coworkers, and is something that should be addressed before the final decision to have AGB surgery is made.

Family Stress

You've read repeatedly in this book that obesity is a disease. When confronted with other diseases such as cancer or heart problems, families seem to be drawn together to face the adversity. "Mom has cancer!" or "Dad has had a heart attack!" are family rallying cries. So why is it that obesity, and bariatric surgery specifically, often divide families rather than unite them?

There are a number of possible explanations. First, your family member didn't all of a sudden contract obesity. They've had it for years, so what's the big deal now? Second, despite all evidence to the contrary, most people still believe that obesity is a self-inflicted condition—a choice, not an illness. Finally, since multiple family members often suffer from the same problem, it is not unique. Why should one person receive treatment for something that everyone else seems to be able to live with? It sounds like some more of that "me first" attitude again, doesn't it?

In some families everyone seems to be jockeying for recognition, often oblivious to the needs of those they should be closest to. This can create some major conflicts if one person is suddenly getting all the attention. Considerable resentment and jealousy may develop between sibling and parent or between husband and wife. In short, change causes stress, especially if the relationship is already strained.

Over time these stresses can even reach the breaking point. It is widely recognized that divorce is more common among couples where one partner has undergone bariatric surgery and lost a significant amount of weight. But it is totally illogical to assume that weight loss was the only factor. A far more likely explanation is that relationships that are already damaged simply fail to adjust when subjected to the additional strain.

Before considering bariatric surgery, a prospective patient should have a heart-to-heart conversation with every member of their family. Depending on their level of maturity, even children as young as six should be made to feel that they are a part of the decision. They need the chance to express their fears, which will give you the chance to reassure them. Older children, particularly teenagers, are often less willing to express their concerns. If they are old enough to understand, you should discuss specific health issues with them and your reasons behind your decision to have AGB surgery. At the same time you will need to explain that this is not going to change only the way you eat but also the way the family eats.

You and your spouse should sit down together and discuss how having an AGB in the family is going to affect them and everyone else. In fact, this is the first conversation you should have. One of the most important questions I ask each patient during their initial consultation is what their husband or wife thinks about their having bariatric surgery. Sometimes the answer is obvious by virtue of the fact that the spouse has actually accompanied them to their appointment and is there to provide support. Occasionally, both husband and wife even make joint appointments because they are both potential candidates for the AGB. Generally this is a good thing, because it signals that they are in support of each other right from the start. While that is usually a good thing, it is not always the case, as you'll see later.

It is somewhat unusual to find that a spouse is not supportive of the other spouse's decision to get a band, but every now and then I'll have a patient tell me that their husband or wife doesn't think they should need to resort to something as drastic as bariatric surgery. This may be because they fear the risks of the operation, or perhaps they are just skeptical as to whether the procedure will work. They usually suggest that the patient simply try harder to lose weight through dieting and exercise. Interestingly, I have heard a number of patients say that the reason their spouse objects is that they fear they will leave them for someone else after they lose weight.

In addition, family members are often unfamiliar with the AGB procedure and the program that goes along with it. They tend to become more supportive once they have a better understanding of the whole program. To help this process along, I encourage every patient to bring their spouse with them to one of our support group meetings before their surgery. The contacts they make and the stories they hear are usually enough to change the mind of even the most cynical of partners. Gaining their support is an important part of preparing the patient.

Providing Support as a Spouse

If you are the husband or wife of an AGB patient, throughout this book you've read about changes in thought and changes in behavior that ultimately change the patient's life. While I may have made it seem like these changes occur only to the person who has the band, that is far from true. Everyone around them will experience change to one degree or another, and as their spouse you will be affected most of all. The changes you will be asked to make are likely to cause you to become more than just a little uncomfortable.

You will, out of necessity, eat differently. You may also be compelled to exercise, and you'll probably lose some weight yourself. These facts may make you less than excited about your spouse having AGB surgery. But, if you think about it, you should welcome these changes as positive side effects for yourself. Here's a chance to make many of the changes that you have been meaning to make to improve your own health. If you choose to fight these changes, the result will be to slow or even reverse your spouse's progress. And you will likely add to the stress both of you endure in the process.

It isn't always easy to be the supporter in the relationship, but for a while that is likely the way it will seem. Most husbands and wives are enthusiastic supporters of their spouse's efforts, but even if you are their biggest "cheerleader" you will occasionally say or do something that your partner will perceive negatively. Try to avoid anything that could be interpreted as judgmental or critical, especially during the first few weeks after surgery and immediately after an adjustment.

Your spouse will be especially sensitive to almost anything you say during those times. Understand before you say something that your husband or wife is likely to be feeling pretty insecure about the whole process. They don't want to disappoint you or others around them, and they remain uncertain not only of their own success but also of whether the things they are experiencing both physically and emotionally are normal.

In an effort to minimize the damage, the first thing you need to do is dedicate yourself to being a better listener. Nothing says you care more than spending time just listening. Women especially like to have someone to talk to, and one of the most common complaints they have about their husbands is that they don't listen. By the way, if you jumble the letters in the word "listen" you can make another six-letter word that is very closely related. That word is "silent." It is very hard to listen when you are doing all the talking.

One of the things that band patients are particularly sensitive about is spitting up, particularly during meals. They are often extremely embarrassed by it and may even refuse to eat with the rest of the family because they're afraid that they won't be able to control it. Almost anything that you say during an episode of spitting up will be viewed as either critical or patronizing. Even an off-hand gesture can be interpreted as disgust or frustration.

What your banded partner needs is encouragement. Let him or her know that you understand the extremely challenging process of learning to eat differently. One thing you can do to demonstrate your understanding of their situation is to change your own eating style. It is very difficult to accept the idea of always being the last one at the table still eating. You should make a special effort to slow down and take smaller bites. When you finish eating, stay at the table until your partner has also finished. If he or she gets up and goes to the bathroom to spit up something they ate, don't assume they are finished. They will likely be back, and you will be sending the wrong message if they come back to an empty table.

Husbands can send an especially powerful and supportive message to their wives that are struggling to adjust to the band. Just by doing something simple without being asked, such as cleaning up in the kitchen or offering to fix dinner, you will let them know you understand what they are going through and want to help. Whatever you do, don't go running after your spouse to help them in the bathroom. They not only don't need your help, they don't want you to witness the process.

Along that same line, you need to recognize that there are certain foods that almost all band patients have trouble with, such as steaks and chops, as well as most kinds of bread. If you insist on always going out to your favorite steakhouse, your spouse is going to get pretty tired of the shrimp cocktail and the soup of the day. Seafood, chicken, and pasta generally go down much more easily than red meats. And while you're out to dinner, remember that alcohol has more calories than any other food. Don't order a bottle of wine with dinner unless you plan to drink it all. Your partner doesn't need the extra calories and should not be drinking while they eat, so try not to add any unnecessary temptation.

Getting regular exercise is critical to the success of every AGB patient, and that often represents a major lifestyle change. A person who may have been more or less sedentary for many years is likely to require a lot of encouragement when they start an exercise program. That doesn't, however, mean you should go out and buy a family membership at the local fitness center. In fact, doing so may backfire on you.

Extremely obese people are often intimidated by those types of facilities and see themselves as being totally out of place. They frequently sense that all of those slim and trim people are watching them while they struggle just to stay on the treadmill. In some cases it doesn't matter how much you encourage them, they simply won't go.

The better solution is to offer to exercise or at least to walk with them. Everyone enjoys walking more if they have a partner, and it will give you regularly scheduled quality time together. Notice that I said regularly scheduled. If you don't schedule a time for exercise, it simply won't happen. So make it a priority in your own schedule, not just a once-in-a-while effort. Your spouse will feed off your example.

The Enabler

Generally the term "enabler" is used to describe someone who supports the addiction of another person. Whether it's a drug or alcohol addiction or compulsive behaviors like gambling, the enabler helps keep it going. Obesity is really no different. It's an addiction to eating, and most morbidly obese people have one or more enablers in their circle of friends and family who make it easier for them to continue those behaviors that contribute to their weight problem. Experts will tell you that trying to help any addict "kick the habit" is extremely difficult unless you also address the enabler. So, for any patient to be successful, it is necessary for their enablers to recognize their role and become agents for change.

It has been my experience that every band patient goes through times of doubt and frustration, and not uncommonly these feelings manifest themselves as anger or withdrawal. Your natural reaction will very likely be one of sympathy. Sympathy may lead you to some form of pampering to express the fact that you care about them and don't like to see them hurting.

But pampering will only serve to verify their feeling of being a victim of some cruel torture test. If they get enough pampering, the patient will continue those behaviors that generated the sympathy rather than pursuing the new lifestyle goals they previously committed to. If you provide sympathy and pampering, your role will quickly deteriorate into that of an enabler.

Don't misinterpret this idea of withholding sympathy as a license to be unkind. That is not what I'm saying at all. It's important to make a distinction here between sympathy and compassion, and between pampering and caring. It is critical for your band patient to feel as though you care about their struggles and that you have compassion for them as they strive to adapt to a totally unfamiliar situation. Only then will they be comfortable sharing their problems and fears with you and others who are close to them.

Once again, this is a place where you need to be a good listener, not a bunch of advice. They also need for you to be honest with them. It's okay to tell them if you believe their behavior is sabotaging their original plan, but do so with compassion. And no matter what, you need to stand firmly behind them, providing encouragement and re-emphasizing the importance of their primary commitment. That is the best way to demonstrate your compassion and caring spirit.

None of this is going to be easy. The whole process of providing appropriate support may feel foreign to you until you've done it for a while. So, to help you get started, I would recommend that you have an open discussion with the band patient regarding your role in the process before any crisis occurs. Be proactive. Let them know how you intend to support them, and get them to agree with your approach in advance. When the time comes for you to take on the role of "plan advocate," you can do so without feeling guilty. Having a game plan for those difficult times that are bound to come is the surest way to avoid becoming an enabler of destructive behavior.

What Can We Do to Help?

G. Dick Miller, Psychologist

I took a handicapped friend out to dinner. My handicapped friend is gaining weight. And his health is seriously deteriorating because of problems with his brain, a condition aggravated by the weight gain. Other people went with us, and we all know about our handicapped friend's problem.

So what did the people who came along do? First of all, the group insisted on going to dinner at a place known exclusively for its huge, family-style portions of fried chicken, mashed potatoes, and home-baked rolls with butter and honey. When we got there, the dinner conversation started with taking a cooking course. Then it shifted to the new specialty grocery store that had just opened and the variety of foods we "love" there—foods "to die for."

I watched this dynamic and my stomach twisted. We were romanticizing food in the presence of someone we know is killing himself with the stuff. And while the new grocery store is beautiful and a fun place to visit for those who don't suffer weight issues, all this talk about food felt to me like we were talking about how great a recent cocaine snort was to someone who is trying to get off drugs.

I am aware that band patients will have to learn to deal with these and other social scenarios. But what I'm saying is that I'm not a friend to someone who is working to lose weight if I romanticize food with my language. I'm not helping if I insist on taking them to places where the food will tempt them to do things that are not in their best interest. Bringing them food that isn't in their best interest would also fit into the not helping category.

Some band patients are still obsessed with food and haven't dealt with the core issues driving them. It's going to take them some time to adjust. During that process, I don't have to police them, check up on them, or keep track of what and when they're eating. It would be in my best interest and theirs for me to "Let go and let God" (to borrow a slogan from the AA 12-Step program).

There are other ways I can help. I can change the way I talk so I'm not talking about food in tempting ways. I can suggest social activities that don't hinge on food. And I can find gifts or ways to express I care that don't involve food. If I want to help, I can treat food like the fuel it is, and stop being part of the process of enticement that had a big part of leading the person I care about into problems.

In changing myself, I may experience uncomfortable self-talk, some awkwardness as I try new things, some discomfort and inconvenience. The band person is going through these same things, and I'll tell you what I tell them. It's going to take some getting used to, and it's necessary to tolerate the discomfort in order to make any kind of change. But frankly, you'll not only be helping the band patient; you'll do yourself a favor, too.

The Band Couple

Earlier I mentioned that both husband and wife undergoing AGB surgery around the same time can be a good thing. They can provide compassion based on their own experience. However, "doing the band together" can also create some big problems. I would never recommend that the procedures be performed on the same day. If a postoperative problem were to develop with either patient, they could potentially need the undivided attention of their spouse. Even if there were no problems, it is still necessary to have someone around who isn't trying to recover from surgery.

I usually recommend waiting at least a week between procedures, and longer if possible. If your partner decides to get a band, please don't make the decision to get one, too, just to make things easier for them. That is a recipe for failure for both of you. Even if you are thoroughly committed to the band for yourself, I would still recommend that you wait until you are reasonably sure how your spouse is going to adapt to the band before going ahead with your own surgery.

The real problems with both partners getting an AGB at the same time occur when they are not equally dedicated to the process. If one is only half-heartedly committed to making the necessary lifestyle changes, their behavior will gradually undermine the efforts of the other. That is certainly not unique to AGB patients and weight-loss efforts.

If a couple decides to quite smoking at the same time, their collective commitment will last only as long as they both remain smoke free. As soon as one starts smoking again, the other is almost certain to follow. If either partner becomes unmotivated, eventually they both become coenablers.

Tynele's Story

My husband, his mom, and his sister all have bands, and I watched their progress as a bystander until I got a band myself two years ago. It has been different, that's for sure, and my little bit of progress hasn't come without a price.

I remember my husband got discouraged, and I thought he was impatient. But now I realize that there's a discouragement phase between the time you get a band and the time you see real progress. I lived in that place for quite a while.

I started at 306 and am now at 240 in two years. I remember how especially slow it seemed in the beginning. I lost 16 pounds pre-op, and at my six-week post-op appointment I'd lost only 2 more for a total of 18 pounds. At three months I was barely at minus 20 pounds. Back then, when I weighed in, I'd be up 1 or 2 pounds and the next time down 1 or 2. I do everything I'm supposed to. I don't drink with meals, I exercise with my husband, I drink water instead of soda, and I cut out between-meal snacks.

My husband has lost 166 pounds in just over a year. And I am pleased to talk about his weight loss. But my coworkers are band people and my family members have bands, and since at three months I'd lost only 20 pounds, I felt I wasn't doing well by comparison. Back then, I hated for people to ask about me. I tried to say, "I'm doing great," but people would press me for the actual pounds. When they heard my meager progress, I thought they assumed I was doing something wrong.

Right at first I had a lot of fills. And that was discouraging. I was hungry again two weeks post-op, like I didn't have a band. The first fill I couldn't feel any difference. The second one I barely felt a difference, and the same with the third and the fourth. I finally got a fill I feel comfortable with. I have never thrown up, although I have experienced the discomfort of food getting stuck because of too big a bite or not chewing enough.

There are big differences from watching someone with a band and having one myself. I've gained an appreciation for what band people go through. I remember thinking when I'd see my husband struggle with his food, "Why don't you just take a smaller bite?" But I found I had trouble adjusting to smaller bites, too. And it's more than just cutting the food into smaller pieces. I've found it's hard for me to chew enough even if I take smaller bites.

I exercise with my husband, but I was used to being the healthier one. Now he's catching up. He can outwalk me, and he couldn't a year ago.

Of course, now I notice a lot of positive differences at minus 66 pounds. Right before surgery my knees started hurting, and now they don't. We live in a hilly place and we can both walk the hills, no problem, when we couldn't before. But the most encouraging thing for me was getting remeasured. When I told the dietician I was discouraged about my progress, she told me that she encourages band patients to be measured at 3, 6, 9, and 12 months post-op. I was reluctant. But the difference in inches was surprising. I lost 3.25 inches in my upper arm alone, and that's a spot I'm concerned about. I'm one of the youngest band patients I know, and I have decided the best thing about losing so gradually is my skin has a chance to adjust.

Despite my discouragement in the beginning, I have no regrets. Even up to the day of surgery, I thought, "Am I doing the right thing?" As soon as I woke up I knew I'd made a positive change, and I still think so. And now my husband and I are trying to have a baby, which is something we've both always wanted.

The Physical Changes

You need to recognize the fact that band patients get caught up in the numbers. They generally measure their success only in terms of pounds lost, or a closely related measurement such as dress size for women and pant size for men. Part of your job is to acknowledge changes in those numbers when they share them with you and provide an element of praise.

Everybody likes to be congratulated when they do something positive, and that is particularly true when it comes to weight loss. You should remember to take advantage of every opportunity for praise. You might even want to have little celebrations whenever certain milestones are reached. Just don't send candy; it might sound good, but it sends the wrong message.

Every band patient gets excited about buying a smaller dress or a smaller belt, as the case may be. When your wife or husband comes home with a new purchase, seize the opportunity to make a fuss over their recent success. But, husbands, just a word of caution! Don't ask the size of that new dress. If she wants you to know, she'll tell you. Talking about women's dress sizes can be a very slippery slope for guys. You should just acknowledge that she looks great and leave it at that.

It can also be tempting to buy clothing for your spouse, but be careful. If you buy it too small, they'll think you are disappointed in their progress. If you buy it too big, you're in even more trouble. If you want to be safe, you should probably just give a gift card and let them pick out something for themselves.

Along with changes in weight and size come renewed energy levels and physical capabilities. I have had many patients tell me after losing only 20 or 30 pounds that they are now able to do things with their family that were previously not possible. They relate being able to go shopping at the mall, swimming with their kids, and even taking a hiking trip.

This raises the question, Should you actively look for things that you can now do together? The answer is both yes and no. You should not be afraid to ask whether they would like to join you in any activity, but don't assume that their answer will always be yes. They may still be uncertain of how much they can actually do. Whatever you do, don't plan a surprise camping trip in the mountains, or something similar, until you are certain that your spouse is not only capable but also would be excited about such a trip. If the activity you have planned ends up being beyond their capability, they will assume that they have disappointed you. That will likely discourage both of you from undertaking future activities together.

I frequently get asked whether there are any physical restrictions when a person has an AGB. The short answer is no, none that I am aware of. I have had patients ride horses and motorcycles, run marathons, and scuba dive following AGB surgery. Obviously, no major physical activity should be undertaken until the surgical wounds are completely healed—usually a couple of weeks. But before you drag your spouse out into the ocean for a dive to 60 feet, I would suggest that you ask their surgeon about whatever activity you may have planned. You also need to make sure that both of you are physically fit enough to take on the planned activity.

Renewed interest in sexual activity is also common in both men and women who lose weight and regain their positive self-image. While this can be a source of mutual enjoyment, like the other changes we've discussed, it is likely to be a gradual process. Once again, the best way to deal with this subject is to have an open and honest dialog between you and your partner. You may even want to use the fact that this subject was mentioned in this book as a graceful means of starting the conversation. When you do, remember that although your spouse may have changed physically, he or she is still likely to be experiencing a significant amount of emotional stress. Depending on how long it has been since they last experienced sexual intimacy, it may take a while before they are comfortable.

Along with a renewed interest in sexual activity, many young AGB patients also experience an increase in fertility. Morbid obesity is a common cause of menstrual irregularities and failure to ovulate in women, as well as low sperm counts in men. Weight loss can often improve these problems, allowing previously infertile couples to become pregnant. A woman who is in her childbearing years should consult with an obstetrician/gynecologist regarding her ability as well as the advisability of becoming pregnant, whether she is the band patient or her husband is the one losing weight. Obviously, not everyone who loses weight is able to get pregnant, but for those who are, it can be one of the greatest benefits of weight loss they will ever receive.

While successful weight loss often improves self-esteem, the excess saggy skin that results from shrinking fat stores can profoundly damage some people's self-image. Because the early excitement is always based on pounds lost, this side effect is often overlooked by others, but not by the patient. In response to a compliment about how good she looked after losing nearly 100 pounds, one patient said, "You should see me naked!"

When your spouse asks whether you think they look older because of their hanging chin or other sagging parts, you will need to be particularly tactful. Your response should be along the lines of, "Well, we knew all along that with your successful weight loss the skin might seem a little lose in some areas."

This is a plain vanilla answer, so as you are saying the words you should anticipate a follow-up question. "Do you think I should have plastic surgery?" Now they are getting to the heart of the matter. You should recognize that, like any subjective question, there is no right answer. If you say yes, then you've not only given your approval, you've also indirectly implied that you don't like the way he or she looks now. If you say no, then you come across as not caring or perhaps just cheap!

A subjective question requires a subjective and diplomatic answer. Try simply rephrasing the question with a response such as "I think you look great just the way you are, but if you feel strongly about it and you want to look into your options, that's okay with me." In this way you are neither agreeing nor disagreeing. Instead you have empowered your partner. You've given your permission to get more information.

Conclusion

Learning to live with someone who has a band sounds like a terribly arduous task. However, for most spouses and family members, it turns into a true labor of love. The feeling you will have as you watch your husband or wife, or your mom or dad, emerge from a lifetime of obesity is worth whatever sacrifice you are asked to make.

What's more, once you realize that obesity is a disease that can be conquered, and that you can play a significant role in that effort, you won't see it as something that you have to do. You'll see it as something you have the privilege of doing.

Resources

Body Mass Index (BMI) Information

Body Mass Index (BMI) Categories for Obesity

BMI	Category
25 to 30	Overweight
Over 30 to 40	Obese
Over 40 to 80	Morbidly Obese
Over 80	Super Obese

Determine your BMI by taking your weight in pounds and your height in inches and finding your corresponding BMI on the table on the following page.

Books and Publications

Eating Well After Weight Loss Surgery by Patt Levine

Fit From Within: 101 Simple Secrets to Change Your Body and Your Life by Victoria Moran; a series of essays aimed at helping forge a new relationship with food, exercise, our bodies, and our lives.

Laparoscopic Adjustable Gastric Banding by Jessie H. Ahroni, Ph.D., A.R.N.P.

LAP-BAND® for Life by Ariel Ortiz Lagardere, M.D., F.A.C.S.

Online Support Groups

Bandsters
health.groups.yahoo.com/group/Bandsters/
For those who have had or are considering band surgery.

Smart Bandsters
health.groups.yahoo.com/group/SmartBandsters/
For those who have had or are considering band surgery, or who already have a band.

Body Mass Index (BMI) Table

Height in Inches

Weight in Pounds	60	61	62	63	64	65	66	67	68	69	70	71	72	73	74	75	76
150	29.3	28.3	27.4	26.6	25.7	25.0	24.2	23.5	22.8	22.2	21.5	20.9	20.3	19.8	19.3	18.7	18.3
155	30.3	29.3	28.4	27.5	26.6	25.8	25.0	24.3	23.6	22.9	22.2	21.6	21.0	20.4	19.9	19.4	18.9
160	31.2	30.2	29.3	28.3	27.5	26.6	25.8	25.1	24.3	23.6	23.0	22.3	21.7	21.1	20.5	20.0	19.5
165	32.2	31.2	30.2	29.2	28.3	27.5	26.6	25.8	25.1	24.4	23.7	23.0	22.4	21.8	21.2	20.6	20.1
170	33.2	32.1	31.1	30.1	29.2	28.3	27.4	26.6	25.8	25.1	24.4	23.7	23.1	22.4	21.8	21.2	20.7
175	34.2	33.1	32.0	31.0	30.1	29.1	28.2	27.4	26.6	25.8	25.1	24.4	23.7	23.1	22.5	21.9	21.3
180	35.2	34.0	32.9	31.9	30.9	30.0	29.1	28.2	27.4	26.6	25.8	25.1	24.4	23.7	23.1	22.5	21.9
185	36.1	35.0	33.8	32.8	31.8	30.8	29.9	29.0	28.1	27.3	26.5	25.8	25.1	24.4	23.8	23.1	22.5
190	37.1	35.9	34.8	33.7	32.6	31.6	30.7	29.8	28.9	28.1	27.3	26.5	25.8	25.1	24.4	23.7	23.1
195	38.1	36.8	35.7	34.5	33.5	32.4	31.5	30.5	29.6	28.8	28.0	27.2	26.4	25.7	25.0	24.4	23.7
200	39.1	37.8	36.6	35.4	34.3	33.3	32.3	31.3	30.4	29.5	28.7	27.9	27.1	26.4	25.7	25.0	24.3
205	40.0	38.7	37.5	36.3	35.2	34.1	33.1	32.1	31.2	30.3	29.4	28.6	27.8	27.0	26.3	25.6	25.0
210	41.0	39.7	38.4	37.2	36.0	34.9	33.9	32.9	31.9	31.0	30.1	29.3	28.5	27.7	27.0	26.2	25.6
215	42.0	40.6	39.3	38.1	36.9	35.8	34.7	33.7	32.7	31.8	30.8	30.0	29.2	28.4	27.6	26.9	26.2
220	43.0	41.6	40.2	39.0	37.8	36.6	35.5	34.5	33.5	32.5	31.6	30.7	29.8	29.0	28.2	27.5	26.8
225	43.9	42.5	41.2	39.9	38.6	37.4	36.3	35.2	34.2	33.2	32.3	31.4	30.5	29.7	28.9	28.1	27.4
230	44.9	43.5	42.1	40.7	39.5	38.3	37.1	36.0	35.0	34.0	33.0	32.1	31.2	30.3	29.5	28.7	28.0
235	45.9	44.4	43.0	41.6	40.3	39.1	37.9	36.8	35.7	34.7	33.7	32.8	31.9	31.0	30.2	29.4	28.6
240	46.9	45.3	43.9	42.5	41.2	39.9	38.7	37.6	36.5	35.4	34.4	33.5	32.6	31.7	30.8	30.0	29.2
245	47.8	46.3	44.8	43.4	42.1	40.8	39.5	38.4	37.3	36.2	35.2	34.2	33.2	32.3	31.5	30.6	29.8
250	48.8	47.2	45.7	44.3	42.9	41.6	40.4	39.2	38.0	36.9	35.9	34.9	33.9	33.0	32.1	31.2	30.4
260	50.8	49.1	47.6	46.1	44.6	43.3	42.0	40.7	39.5	38.4	37.3	36.3	35.3	34.3	33.4	32.5	31.6
270	52.7	51.0	49.4	47.8	46.3	44.9	43.6	42.3	41.1	39.9	38.7	37.7	36.6	35.6	34.7	33.7	32.9
280	54.7	52.9	51.2	49.6	48.1	46.6	45.2	43.9	42.6	41.3	40.2	39.1	38.0	36.9	36.0	35.0	34.1
290	56.6	54.8	53.0	51.4	49.8	48.3	46.8	45.4	44.1	42.8	41.6	40.4	39.3	38.3	37.2	36.2	35.3
300	58.6	56.7	54.9	53.1	51.5	49.9	48.4	47.0	45.6	44.3	43.0	41.8	40.7	39.6	38.5	37.5	36.5
310	60.5	58.6	56.7	54.9	53.2	51.6	50.0	48.6	47.1	45.8	44.5	43.2	42.0	40.9	39.8	38.7	37.7
320	62.5	60.5	58.5	56.7	54.9	53.3	51.6	50.1	48.7	47.3	45.9	44.6	43.4	42.2	41.1	40.0	39.0
330	64.4	62.4	60.4	58.5	56.6	54.9	53.3	51.7	50.2	48.7	47.4	46.0	44.8	43.5	42.4	41.2	40.2
340	66.4	64.2	62.2	60.2	58.4	56.6	54.9	53.3	51.7	50.2	48.8	47.4	46.1	44.9	43.7	42.5	41.4
350	68.4	66.1	64.0	62.0	60.1	58.2	56.5	54.8	53.2	51.7	50.2	48.8	47.5	46.2	44.9	43.7	42.6
360	70.3	68.0	65.8	63.8	61.8	59.9	58.1	56.4	54.7	53.2	51.7	50.2	48.8	47.5	46.2	45.0	43.8
370	72.3	69.9	67.7	65.5	63.5	61.6	59.7	58.0	56.3	54.6	53.1	51.6	50.2	48.8	47.5	46.2	45.0
380	74.2	71.8	69.5	67.3	65.2	63.2	61.3	59.5	57.8	56.1	54.5	53.0	51.5	50.1	48.8	47.5	46.3
390	76.2	73.7	71.3	69.1	66.9	64.9	62.9	61.1	59.3	57.6	56.0	54.4	52.9	51.5	50.1	48.7	47.5
400	78.1	75.6	73.2	70.9	68.7	66.6	64.6	62.6	60.8	59.1	57.4	55.8	54.3	52.8	51.4	50.0	48.7
420	82.0	79.4	76.8	74.4	72.1	69.9	67.8	65.8	63.9	62.0	60.3	58.6	57.0	55.4	53.9	52.5	51.1
440	85.9	83.1	80.5	77.9	75.5	73.2	71.0	68.9	66.9	65.0	63.1	61.4	59.7	58.1	56.5	55.0	53.6
460	89.8	86.9	84.1	81.5	79.0	76.5	74.2	72.0	69.9	67.9	66.0	64.2	62.4	60.7	59.1	57.5	56.0
480	93.7	90.7	87.8	85.0	82.4	79.9	77.5	75.2	73.0	70.9	68.9	66.9	65.1	63.3	61.6	60.0	58.4
500	97.7	94.5	91.5	88.6	85.8	83.2	80.7	78.3	76.0	73.8	71.7	69.7	67.8	66.0	64.2	62.5	60.9

Legend:
- □ Normal
- ▨ Obese
- ▨ Morbidly Obese
- ▨ Super Obese

Source: Master Center for Minimally Invasive Surgery, Texas, LLP.

Websites

American Board of Plastic Surgery website
www.abplsurg.org
Offers information on choosing a surgeon and answers to frequently asked questions.

American Society of General Surgeons
www.theasgs.org
Offers information on the PALSS certification of laparoscopic surgical skills.

American Society of Plastic Surgeons
www.plasticsurgery.org
Offers procedure information along with before and after photos.

Body Mass Index (BMI) Calculator
www.nhlbisupport.com/bmi/
BMI Calculator provided at the National Heart, Lung and Blood Institute website and sponsored by the National Institutes of Health.

Diet Facts
DietFacts.com
Nutrition facts for foods, including fast food and popular restaurants.

Fit Day
FitDay.com
An online diet and fitness journal. Especially helpful in determining individual protein and calorie intake needs.

WLS Lifestyles Magazine Online
www.wlslifestyles.com
A magazine aimed at inspiring, educating, and supporting life after weight-loss surgery.

Glossary

Abdominoplasty   Also known as the "tummy tuck," this plastic surgery procedure involves removal of excess skin and tightening of the abdominal area.

Adipose tissue   The medical term for stored fat.

Adjustable Gastric Banding (AGB)   This is the generic term for the banding process, including both the Lap Band® and Obtech banding systems.

Alimentary tract   The main component of the digestive system, consisting of a long tube that begins at the mouth and ends at the anus.

American Board of Plastic Surgery (ABPS)   The recognized national organization responsible for certifying plastic surgeons.

American Society of Bariatric Surgeons (ASBS)   A national organization of surgeons who specialize in the surgical treatment of obesity.

American Society of General Surgeons (ASGS)   A national organization composed of general surgeon specialists.

Amino acids   The small molecules that are bound together to form more complex protein molecules.

Amnesia   The inability to remember an event. Sometimes patients experience a degree of amnesia from just before surgery to well after the event as a result of anesthesia medications.

Amylase   A digestive enzyme secreted by the pancreas and found to a lesser degree in saliva, which breaks down starches and other carbohydrates, converting them into simple sugars that can be absorbed into the bloodstream through the intestine.

Anemia   A condition characterized by fewer than expected red blood cells in the blood. This may be due to blood loss (bleeding), abnormal destruction of red blood cells (hemolytic), or inadequate production of red blood cells as a result of a lack of iron or a deficiency of certain dietary elements such as Vitamin B-12. See Vitamin B-12.

Anesthesia   The administration of specific drugs to block the painful effects of surgery. A medically induced sleeplike state that allows for the safe and controlled performance of surgery.

Anesthesiologist   A physician who specializes in putting patients to sleep for surgery and monitors them during the procedure.

Anesthesiology   The medical specialty of placing people into a sleeplike state or providing other means of pain relief during surgery.

Antibiotic   Any of a variety of medications designed to kill bacteria and aid in the body's efforts to fight infection.

Anticoagulant   A medication used to keep blood from clotting. Commonly referred to as a blood thinner.

Apron   The excess skin of the lower abdomen, which can hang down over the pubic region following weight loss.

Arteriosclerosis   The development of deposits within the walls of arteries resulting in thickening of the arterial walls and narrowing of the arterial channels. Frequently associated with hypertension.

Arthritis   Any condition in which one or more joints become inflamed.

Aspiration   The process of food or fluids passing from the normal swallowing channel into the trachea, or windpipe.

Atelectasis   The collapse of small airways in the lower aspects of the lungs, trapping mucus and bacteria that can turn into pneumonia. Deep breathing and coughing post-op help prevent this condition.

Attention Deficit Hyperactivity Disorder (ADHD)   A psychological disorder characterized by, among other things, an inability to control impulsive behavior.

Band   The generic term for the silastic ring used in the AGB process, including both the Allergan (Inamed or Bioenterics) and Johnson and Johnson (Swedish or Obtech) bands.

Band migration (gastric erosion)   A relatively rare, but serious complication of the adjustable gastric band whereby the band erodes through the wall of the stomach. The erosion may be attributed to the band placing excessive pressure on the stomach and cutting off circulation in the affected areas. It may also be due to ulcers within the stomach penetrating out to connect with the band. The usual remedy is removal of the band.

Band slippage   A condition in which the band around the stomach moves up or more commonly down on the stomach, away from its initial intended position.

Bandster   A person who has undergone the placement of an Adjustable Gastric Band as weight-loss surgery.

Bariatric surgery   The treatment of excess body weight using one of several surgical procedures designed to alter the digestive system in an attempt to promote weight loss.

Bariatrics   The medical specialty that involves the study and treatment of excess body weight.

Barium   A chalky-tasting fluid that is used in a number of X-ray studies to outline the anatomy of parts of the intestinal tract.

Barium swallow   An X-ray study in which barium is used to define the anatomy of the upper digestive tract. This test may be used to demonstrate swallowing abnormalities in the esophagus, band displacement on the upper stomach, reflux of stomach contents into the esophagus, or the presence of a hiatal hernia.

Basal layer   A layer of cells within the skin that separates the top layer, or epidermis, from the bottom layer, or dermis.

Bat wings   The excessive skin hanging from the under side of the upper arms, usually after weight loss.

Belt lipectomy   Removal of excess skin in a circle from the stomach, flanks, and back, and lifting of the skin of the buttocks and the outer aspects of the thighs.

Bile   The yellow to greenish liquid material secreted by the liver through the bile ducts into the small intestine, which is essential to the process of breaking down fatty foods into tiny particles that can be absorbed into the bloodstream during digestion.

Bile ducts   A system of tubes that gather and transport bile from the liver to the intestines.

Biliopancreatic Diversion with Duodenal Switch (BPD-DS)   A complex bariatric operation in which the size of the stomach is reduced via a sleeve gastrectomy; then the duodenum is divided, the outlet of the stomach is connected to the small intestine, and the remaining part of the small intestine is reconnected well downstream, near the end of the ileum. The procedure combines both the restriction of a small gastric pouch and the malabsorption effects of a short intestine.

Biliopancreatic fluid   The combination of bile from the liver and enzymes from the pancreas that are essential for the digestion of fats and carbohydrates.

Bioenterics LAP-BAND®: The LAP-BAND® is an adjustable gastric band that is FDA approved in the United States as a restrictive surgical option for the treatment of serious obesity.

BiPAP   A machine designed to be worn at night to provide airway support during sleep for people with sleep apnea.

Blood glucose   The measurement of the amount of sugar in the blood.

Body contouring   A term used to describe plastic surgical procedures following weight loss that emphasize removing skin or changing the body shape and appearance to more pleasing proportions and removing problem areas.

Body Mass Index (BMI)   A commonly used measurement that combines a person's weight and height. BMI is generally accepted as the standard for determining overweight and obesity diagnoses. The formula for calculating BMI is (weight in kilograms) divided by (height in meters squared).

Canula   A small tube that is placed into the abdominal cavity through the skin and muscular wall during laparoscopic surgery, which acts as a conduit or portal for the introduction of long slender instruments used during surgery.

Cardiac stress test   A group of tests designed to determine how well the heart functions during periods of maximal stress or exertion. One or more of these tests may be performed prior to surgery in an attempt to identify problems that could arise during the stress of anesthesia and an operation.

Cardiology   A branch of medical science having to do with the heart.

Catheter   A tube inserted into the body to serve a medical purpose. One common type of catheter is a urinary catheter, which is placed into the bladder to drain urine.

Cells   The smallest units of living tissue.

Cellulite   Lumpy fat stores under the skin.

Cholecystokinin   A chemical released by the stomach as it fills up with food that stimulates the gallbladder to contract, literally squeezing bile out of the gallbladder, through the main bile duct, and into the intestine, to assist in the digestion of recently ingested fat.

Circumferential body lift   See Belt lipectomy.

Cirrhosis   A scarring of the liver that can interfere with the function of the liver as well as the flow of blood from the intestine through the liver.

Clinical research trials   Research studies designed to evaluate the safety and effectiveness of medications or medical devices by monitoring their effects on large groups of people.

Cognitive dissonance   A pattern of negative thinking generated by the brain that nearly always occurs whenever a person tries a new activity or behavior.

Colon   That portion of the intestinal tract responsible for absorbing most of the water from the waste material left after the digestive process. The colon is also responsible for transporting the waste to the rectum for evacuation in the form of feces.

Comorbidity (Comorbidities)   Serious medical condition(s), usually mentioned as a result of another chronic condition because they compound the problem. For example, high blood pressure is frequently a comorbidity to obesity.

CPAP (Continuous Positive Airway Pressure)   A machine designed to be worn at night by people with sleep apnea to support the upper airways during sleep.

Crohn's disease   A form of inflammatory bowel disease that has no known cause and can influence the risk of gastric surgery, including the placement of an adjustable gastric band.

Deep Vein Thrombosis (DVT)   The clotting of pooled blood in the large veins of the legs and pelvis.

Dehydration   A condition in which the body doesn't have enough water to function normally.

Dermis   The deep layer of the skin, which contains the blood vessels, nerves, and glands of the skin.

Diabetes   A shortened term for diabetes mellitus. See Diabetes mellitus.

Diabetes insipidus   A pathologic condition in which the body loses much of its ability to retain water normally.

Diabetes mellitus   A chronic medical condition affecting the uptake and utilization of glucose by the cells of the body, which requires the presence of insulin produced within the pancreas. The condition may be the result of inadequate insulin production or the development of resistance of cells to available insulin.

Diaphragm   The broad, flat muscle that separates the chest cavity from the abdominal cavity. The diaphragm contracts and relaxes as part of the process of breathing.

Diastolic pressure   The second number in the blood pressure, which is the minimum pressure remaining within the arteries during the period between heartbeats.

Diet   Food and liquids that are taken into the body and subsequently digested within the intestinal tract.

Dietitian   A expert who is trained in the dietary needs and nutrition of the human body and the effects of nutrition on health and disease.

Digestion   The process of breaking food down into its essential components to fuel and provide the basic building blocks for the body. Includes both mechanical and chemical breakdown of food.

Diverticulitis   A condition caused by chronically higher than normal pressure within the colon in an attempt to move very small, very firm stools through for elimination. Often caused by not enough roughage in the diet.

Dumping syndrome   The term used to describe the rapid addition of large volumes of water from the bloodstream into the intestine in direct response to eating a large amount of sugar or carbohydrate. This is common in gastric bypass patients because the stomach normally serves as a buffer, allowing only small amounts of highly concentrated sugar or carbohydrates to reach the intestine at any one time. Symptoms can include sudden crampy abdominal pain, nausea, bloating, diarrhea, lightheadedness, sweating, rapid heart rate, dizziness, and fatigue.

Duodenal Switch (DS)   See Biliopancreatic Diversion with Duodenal Switch (BPD-DS).

Duodenum   The first part of the small intestine, approximately 1 foot long, which begins at the bottom of the stomach and ends at the second part of the small intestine, the jejunum. The duodenum is the point where chemical digestion begins, since this is where bile and pancreas enzymes are added to food.

Early obstruction   A condition in post-op AGB patients whereby the band can be so tight that not even fluids can pass through.

Edema   Swelling caused by an accumulation of water in dependent tissues with poor circulation.

Electrocardiogram   A common test used to determine the electrical activity within the heart, which can suggest possible problems. This test is commonly obtained prior to surgery in patients at risk for cardiac problems.

Electrocautery   A technique that employs electrical current to control bleeding during a surgical procedure.

Emulsification   The process of breaking fatty foods into tiny particles or globules in the stomach during digestion, which requires bile from the liver.

Endoscopic examination   The procedure to examine the inside of the esophagus, stomach, and duodenum. See endoscopy.

Endoscopy   A diagnostic test in which a flexible lighted tube is passed through the mouth, down the esophagus, and into the stomach and duodenum, providing a visual examination for possible problems inside these parts of the digestive tract.

Endotracheal tube   A tube placed through the vocal cords, into the windpipe, or trachea, to maintain breathing during surgery.

Epidermis   The superficial layer of skin composed mostly of dead cells, which are constantly being replaced.

Esophageal hiatus   The natural opening in the diaphragm through which the esophagus passes just prior to emptying into the stomach.

Esophageal varicies   Dilated veins in the lower esophagus that are usually the result of restricted blood flow through the liver; commonly associated with cirrhosis.

Esophagus   The muscular tube that transports food from the back of the throat to the stomach.

Excess Weight Loss (EWL)   The measure of how much weight has been lost in relation to an individual's ideal body weight. This is usually stated as a percentage. For example, a person with an ideal body weight of 150 pounds, who has lost from their actual starting weight of 300 pounds down to 225 pounds, would have a 50 percent EWL (75 lbs. lost / 300 lbs. − 150 lbs.).

Fatty liver   A liver in which too much glycogen is stored, which can potentially interfere with normal liver function.

Fecal material   Roughage that is left over after the digestive process, which is transported through the colon and eliminated from the body as a bowel movement.

Fenfluramine®   The brand name of a drug used to achieve weight loss through appetite suppression. This was a component of Fen-phen®, a compound drug that is no longer available in the United States.

Fen-phen®   A brand-name drug combination of Fenfluramine® and Phentermine® created in the 1990s to promote weight loss. It was later taken off the market because it became linked to the development of a type of valvular heart disease thought to be life threatening.

Fill   The process of using a syringe to inject saline or a similar substance into the subcutaneous port of the AGB to increase the tightness of the band around the stomach. This is the process that allows patients to adjust the pressure of the band, thereby affecting how much food they are able to eat and how quickly the food drops into the lower portion of the stomach.

Fluoroscopy   A video X-ray procedure that makes it possible to see internal organs in motion. This may involve swallowing a barium liquid to observe its progress through the area of band restriction.

Follicle   A specialized structure in the skin that produces a single hair.

Gallbladder   A small pouch off the bile duct located under the liver, which functions as a temporary storage area for bile before it passes into the intestinal tract.

Gallbladder disease   The presence of inflammation of the gallbladder, stones within the gallbladder, or malfunction of the gallbladder, usually associated with abdominal pain or nausea.

Gallbladder sonogram   A diagnostic test to look at the gallbladder using ultra-high frequency sound waves that bounce back off the tissues and are converted into a visual image.

Gallstones   Rocklike formations that can form within the gallbladder as a result of crystallized bile that may require surgical removal of the gallbladder.

Gastric bypass   See Roux-en-Y Gastric Bypass.

Gastric herniation   A condition in which a portion of the stomach from below the band pushes its way up through the band opening.

Gastric reflux   The presence of stomach contents, usually acid, in the lower esophagus, typically the cause of heartburn.

Gastric sleeve   See Sleeve gastrectomy.

Gastric stapling   A bariatric operation that partitions the stomach with staples into a small upper stomach pouch and a larger lower stomach with a narrow opening for food to pass through between the upper and lower areas.

Gastroenterologist   A medical specialist in the field of gastrointestinal diseases as well as liver disorders.

Gastroesophageal Reflux Disease (GERD)   The condition characterized by the abnormal movement of stomach contents, usually acid, up into the esophagus causing heartburn, chest pain, regurgitation of food, and other related symptoms.

Gastroplasty   Any surgical alteration of the stomach, typically to decrease the size of the stomach. These procedures include various operations including the vertical banded gastroplasty (VGB).

GERD   See gastroesophageal reflux disease.

Glucose   A simple sugar molecule that is a basic component of all starches and complex sugars.

Glycogen   A complex sugar that is produced by the liver from excess glucose and that is stored in the liver for later use when glucose levels in the blood go down and the cells need energy.

Hardening of the arteries   See Arteriosclerosis.

Heat stroke   A condition that occurs when body temperature rises uncontrollably, frequently associated with dehydration.

Heparin   A common anticoagulant or blood thinner, generally given prior to surgery and usually for 12 to 24 hours afterward to prevent deep vein thrombosis and pulmonary embolus.

Hepatic cirrhosis   See Cirrhosis.

Hepatologist A medical doctor who specializes in the diagnosis and treatment of liver diseases.

Hiatal hernia A condition in which the natural opening in the diaphragm, called the esophageal hiatus, becomes stretched, allowing the pressure in the abdomen to push the stomach and other abdominal organs up through this opening into the chest.

HIDA scan A test used to assess the functional capability of the gallbladder. Typically used to determine whether the gallbladder is emptying bile as it should.

High blood pressure A medical condition characterized by consistently elevated pressure within the arteries of the body.

Hydrochloric acid The type of acid produced by the stomach for digestion.

Hypertension See high blood pressure.

Ileum The second half of the small intestine, extending from the midway point to the end of the small intestine, where it empties into the colon.

Incisional hernia A complication of any abdominal operation, more common following open incisions, whereby the muscular layer of the abdominal wall fails to heal completely, allowing the edges of the muscle to separate, creating a defect in the abdominal wall.

Intertriginous moniliasis An infection of the skin caused by the growth of fungus attracted to a warm, moist, and dark place such as under deep folds of skin.

Intestinal bypass See Jejuno-ileal bypass.

Intravenous The injection of medications or fluids directly into the bloodstream through a small catheter placed into a vein.

Intubations A part of the induction of anesthesia that involves placing a tube into the trachea for breathing during surgery.

Jejuno-ileal bypass An older bariatric operation that has not been performed for many years because of the high risk of medical problems associated with the procedure. Also known as JI bypass or intestinal bypass, this surgical procedure shortens the small intestine from its usual length of about 18 feet to only about 4 feet in order to minimize the absorption of food.

Jejunum The second part of the small intestine, starting at the end of the duodenum and ending at the ileum, comprising approximately half of the overall length of the small intestine.

JI bypass See Jejuno-ileal bypass.

Lap Abbreviation for laparoscopic.

Laparoscope A long, thin telescope attached to a high-intensity light source and a miniature video camera that is inserted into the body during laparoscopic surgery to view the working area.

Laparoscopic surgery A minimally invasive surgical technique that involves using cameras and instruments inserted into the body through a number of small incisions rather than the large, open incision common to traditional surgery. Advantages include less pain, faster recovery, and less noticeable scars.

Laparoscopy See Laparoscopic surgery.

Laparotomy An abdominal operation performed through a large incision, allowing the surgeon open access to the abdominal cavity.

LAP-BAND® The trade name for the adjustable gastric band manufactured by Allergan, Inc., formerly Inamed, Inc., and BioEnterics.

Large intestine See Colon.

Leaking band The loss of fluid from the band system, which can either be small and slow or rapid and dramatic. A leak can occur from the injection port, the tubing, or the band itself. Treatments can range from more frequent fills to removal and replacement of the entire band.

Lipase A digestive enzyme produced by the pancreas that works on ingested fatty substances, breaking them down to fatty acids, cholesterol, and other absorbable fat molecules.

Lipids Fatty substances contained in various foods.

Liquid diet A diet that consists of liquids only. No solid foods are permitted. This is often prescribed from one to four weeks following gastric surgery.

Liver The largest solid organ in the abdomen, which is responsible for many vital functions, including making and secreting bile into the alimentary tract, detoxifying blood from the intestine before absorbed nutrients are sent into the bloodstream, and storage of glucose as glycogen for immediate use by the body.

Malabsorptive bariatric procedures Operations designed to remove or change the digestive system in order to interfere with the absorption of nutrients by the intestine.

Malignant An aggressive behavior commonly used to describe cancerous growths.

Melanin The pigment found in the basal layer of the skin, which is responsible for the color of the skin.

Melanocytes The cells present in the basal layer of the skin which produce melanin.

Melanoma An aggressive form of skin cancer arising from melanocytes.

Meridia®   A brand name drug with appetite suppressant and metabolic stimulant properties used to promote weight loss.

Morbidity   A diseased condition or state, the incidence of a disease, or of all diseases in a population. For our purposes, the term can be used either in regard to complications arising from the AGB process or obesity itself.

Morbidly obese   Individuals whose BMI is 40 kg/m² or higher.

Mortality rate   The likelihood of death as a consequence of a particular procedure or treatment. The ratio of the total number of deaths to the total number of procedures or treatments performed. May also be used to describe the likelihood of death because of a particular illness.

Motility   The ability of a part of the intestinal tract to push food from one area to the next using spontaneous motion, a process called peristalsis.

National Institutes of Health (NIH)   A part of the U.S. Department of Health and Human Services and the primary federal agency responsible for conducting and supporting medical research.

Nephrologist   A medical specialist in diseases and disorders of the kidney.

Non-scale Victories (NSVs)   Important milestones during the weight-loss process that represent positive life changes yet don't have to do specifically with weight as measured by the scale.

Non-Steroid Anti-Inflammatory Drugs (NSAIDs)   A large group of drugs that have anti-inflammatory characteristics and that work by inhibiting the production of prostaglandins. Common examples include ibuprofen, ketoprofen, piroxicam, naproxen, aspirin, fenoprofen, indomethacin, and tolmetin. There are many others in this group, and most surgeons recommend they be avoided following AGB or other bariatric procedures, as they may irritate the stomach lining causing ulcerations and even bleeding.

Obese   Those patients with a body mass index over 30 kg/m² but less than 40 kg/m².

Obesity   The medical condition characterized by excess body fat.

Obtech Swedish Adjustable Gastric Band   The adjustable gastric band manufactured by a division of Johnson and Johnson (formerly by Obtech). This is considered a low-pressure band that typically requires more fluid to exert pressure on the stomach.

Operative laparoscopy   See Laparoscopic surgery.

PACU   The postanesthesia care unit, also known as the recovery room.

Pancreas   An organ located behind the stomach that produces the digestive enzymes amylase and lipase, and also contains specialized groups of cells (Islets of Langerhan) that produce insulin.

Panniculectomy   The removal of the pannus, or the "apron," which is the large, hanging skin area at the bottom of the abdomen.

Pannus   The large abdominal "apron" made by the skin that often results when obese patients lose weight.

Peripheral vascular disease   See Arteriosclerosis.

Peristalsis   The process by which the intestinal tract "milks" food and fluid along from one area to the next.

Phenteramine®   A drug used to promote weight loss by acting as an appetite suppressant.

Pickwickian syndrome   A condition named for a character in the Charles Dickens novel *Pickwick Papers* who was extremely obese and would frequently stop breathing as a result of his weight.

Pilo-erector muscle   A tiny muscle attached to the hair follicle that contracts to make the hair stand up.

Plastic surgery   Surgery for the restoration, repair, or reconstruction of body structures.

Plateau   A period of time of two to four weeks, during which an individual who is attempting to lose weight seems to stop losing and remains stable despite continued efforts.

Port   The part of the band system that is accessible with a needle through the skin, used to perform adjustments to the AGB.

Pouch   The small "upper stomach" created by the band as it draws the stomach into an hour-glass shape. This is where your food will go after swallowing, where it will slowly pass through into the lower stomach and on through the digestive tract.

Pre-op diet   A two- to three-week preoperative low-fat, low-carbohydrate diet some surgeons have their patients on prior to surgery in an effort to shrink the size of the liver, making band surgery easier and safer.

Preoperative testing   The battery of tests that help to determine the patient's physical health and fitness to undergo surgery. In addition to a detailed diet and health history and examination, as well as a psychological examination, this may include a full blood workup and electrocardiogram, depending on the patient's age, sex, and relative health status.

Productive Burp (PB)   A common description of the regurgitation of food that has recently been swallowed by a band patient, but remains in the esophagus because the upper stomach pouch is full.

Proficiency Assessment of Laparoscopic Surgical Skills (PALSS) A laparoscopic skills certification process offered by the American Society of General Surgeons (ASGS).

Protease A group of digestive enzymes that break down complex protein molecules into their building blocks known as amino acids. These digestive enzymes are produced by the cells that line the inside of the small intestine and are necessary to convert protein into amino acids for absorption into the bloodstream.

Pulmonary embolus A potentially life-threatening condition in which clotted blood breaks away from the wall of a large vein in the pelvis or legs and travels quickly back to the heart and is then pumped up into the lungs, blocking blood flow through the lung tissue.

Pulmonologist A medical specialist in the field of lung function and lung diseases.

Pulse oximeter A monitoring device placed on a patient's finger or ear lobe, both during and after surgery, to continuously measure the amount of oxygen in the blood.

Pylorus The muscular valve at the bottom of the stomach that prevents food from passing out of the stomach until it has been mixed with stomach acid and becomes the consistency of oatmeal.

Redux® The generic name for a weight-loss drug developed in the 1990s and later taken off the market because it became linked to the development of a type of valvular heart disease thought to be life threatening.

Restriction A term used by AGB patients to describe the feeling that limits the amount of food they can eat.

Restrictive bariatric surgical procedures Weight-loss operations that limit the amount of food that can be eaten but do not otherwise alter the digestive process.

Roughage Foods that contain substantial amounts of material that is not digestible and therefore passes through the intestine as waste without being absorbed.

Roux-en-Y (RNY) gastric bypass The creation of a "Y-shaped street." This is the most common form of gastric bypass surgery. The gastrointestinal tract is rearranged by creating a small upper stomach pouch, and the small intestine is divided with the lower portion connected directly to this pouch, effectively bypassing a good portion of the stomach and duodenum. The "Y" is created by reattaching the upper end of the divided small intestine back into the food stream farther down.

Saliva   The fluid produced by the salivary glands in the mouth, which acts as a lubricant that makes the food easier to swallow. Saliva also contains a small amount of amylase, an enzyme that helps digest carbohydrates.

Salivary glands   Glands in the mouth that produce saliva.

Sebaceous gland   A gland associated with hair follicles that produces an oily substance to lubricate both the hair and the surrounding skin.

Sequential Compression Devices (SCDs)   Inflatable leggings that periodically massage the legs to promote normal circulation during periods of inactivity and are used to help prevent venous thrombosis as well as possible pulmonary embolus.

Short-gut syndrome   A potentially fatal medical condition resulting from inadequate length of small intestine to allow for adequate nutrient absorption. This is a common problem following jejuno-ileal bypass and other "bowel-shortening" procedures. Typical symptoms include uncontrollable diarrhea, dehydration, kidney stones, anemia, malnutrition, various vitamin deficiencies, and even liver failure.

Sleep apnea   The result of airway blockage, which occurs during sleep if the tissues of the upper air passages relax, allowing the air passage to collapse. The normal automatic breathing process is interrupted temporarily until the person awakens sufficiently to initiate voluntary breathing. Sleep apnea can severely limit restful sleep.

Sleeve gastrectomy   A restrictive bariatric operation that converts the stomach into a long tube with removal of the remaining portion of the stomach pouch.

Sliming   The result of blockage at the site of the band, causing the production of a large amount of foamy mucus that quickly builds up in the esophagus, which, along with an increase in salivation, is the body's attempt to provide lubrication to remove the obstacle.

Slippage   See Band slippage.

Small bowel limb   The segment of intestine that extends from the stomach down to where the small intestine is reconnected.

Small intestine   That portion of the digestive system that is approximately 18 feet long, where virtually all absorption of nutrients takes place. Tiny molecules of simple sugars, fatty acids, amino acids, vitamins, and minerals are all absorbed into the bloodstream through the lining of the small intestine.

Stoma   An opening from one area of the intestinal tract to another, or to the outside.

Stomach   The large pouch portion of the digestive tract located just below the diaphragm. Normally the stomach can hold a liter or more of food and fluid. It produces a highly concentrated solution of hydrochloric acid, capable of breaking down the structure of even the toughest foods we ingest. And it acts like a big mixer, literally grinding food and mechanically transforming it into a thick paste.

Stomach stapling   See Gastric stapling.

Stool   Waste material from digestion, stored in the colon until eliminated.

Stretch marks   Unsightly, permanent, linear scars in the skin that are the result of the skin's stretching rapidly or beyond its ability to grow.

Subcutaneous adipose tissue   The layer of tissue between the skin and the muscle layers where significant body fat is stored.

Subtotal gastrectomy   A surgical procedure in which most of the stomach is removed.

Sugar diabetes   See Diabetes mellitus.

Super obese   A term used to describe individuals whose BMI is over 80 kg/m^2.

Sweat gland   A gland within the skin that excretes water to help cool the body through the process of evaporation.

Systolic pressure   The first number in a blood pressure reading, which represents the peak pressure that exists when the heart is actively contracting to push blood through the arteries.

Terminal ileum   The very last part of the small intestine, where key vitamins and bile salts are absorbed.

Trachea   The anatomic term for the windpipe, meaning the airway from the back of the throat to the lungs.

Trocar   A surgical instrument with either a sharp triangular point or a tapered point, used to insert a canula through the abdominal wall during laparoscopic surgery.

Tubing   The part of the AGB that connects the port where saline is injected to the band around the stomach.

Tummy tuck   A plastic surgical procedure designed to remove excess skin from the lower part of the abdomen. See Abdominoplasty.

Type 2 diabetes   A medical condition commonly associated with obesity, in which the body's ability to utilize glucose is impaired. This may be due to reduced insulin production but is more often related to the development of resistance to the effects of insulin, necessary for the cellular absorption of glucose from the bloodstream.

Upper GI X-ray A diagnostic test in which the patient is asked to swallow a liquid solution containing barium that shows up on an X-ray, outlining the esophagus, stomach, duodenum, and a portion of the small intestines.

VBG Abbreviation for Vertical Banded Gastroplasty.

Venous stasis ulcers Skin ulcers, most commonly found in the ankle region, caused by chronic edema and poor circulation.

Venous thrombosis A condition in which blood clots within the veins, usually caused by stagnant flow.

Vertical Banded Gastroplasty (VBG) A restrictive bariatric procedure that combines an element of gastric stapling and a fixed, nonadjustable gastric band placed between the small upper pouch and the larger lower stomach.

Villae Tiny fingerlike projections that blanket the inside of the small intestine and that contain a network of capillaries capable of absorbing molecular nutrients directly into the bloodstream.

Villus A single fingerlike structure. See Villae.

Visceral fat deposits Deposits of fat around organs that can interfere with the organ's function, such as fat deposits around the heart.

Vitamin B-12 A vitamin that plays an important role in the process of making red blood cells, which carry oxygen to the body. Vitamin B-12 is also important to normal nerve function.

Windpipe See Trachea.

WLS Abbreviation for weight-loss surgery.

Xenical® A weight-loss drug that binds up ingested fat inside the intestine to prevent it from being absorbed by the digestive system.

Acknowledgments

This book would not have been possible without the continuous effort and resolve of my coauthor Linda Rohrbough. She willingly shared her considerable experience as a professional writer to coach me through the maze of obstacles that cause many "want to be authors" to end up as just that. I also must express my appreciation for the confidence and trust that each and every patient has shown toward me, and my staff, allowing us to help them achieve success. We consider it an honor and a privilege to be of service. A special thanks is owed to those who were willing to share their stories to make this book come alive.

I also need to thank my incredible staff at the MASTER CENTER® for Minimally Invasive Surgery—Tamara Battle, our receptionist; Terri Gregg and Angie Gates, our patient coordinators; Suzanne Jones, our current office manager; Sue Magie, our former office manager; and Stacie Bussey, RNFA, my nurse/first assistant/girl Friday for the last 16 years and constant source of energy. Our program would not be possible if it were not for the devotion of these amazing individuals.

A special thanks goes out to Diane Wallace, our phenomenal dietitian. She has been instrumental in organizing and running the day-to-day activities of our Comprehensive Weight Management Program. But, in addition to her key role as dietitian and personal coach to each patient, she organizes support group meetings, arranges for mentors, produces our monthly newsletter, and collects most of our data, along with a thousand other thankless tasks.

Our clinical psychologists, Drs. Steven Greer and Dick Miller, also deserve individual mention for their critical roles in the psychological assessment and behavior modification aspects of our program, and for their considerable contributions to this book.

Most of all, I want to thank Donna, my wife of 25 years, not only for her constant love and support this past year while I was writing this book but also for those countless hours of patiently waiting for me to come home. To be a surgeon's wife for that long surely makes one eligible for sainthood.

Finally, I know I speak for everyone involved in this project when I say we believe that all things happen for a reason, and God is in fact the author of all things. I only hope that in some small way, our efforts to share the information contained in this book will bring glory to Him.

Robert W. Sewell, M.D.
March 2007
www.MasterCenters.com

I'd like first to acknowledge Dr. Sewell for the foresight to come up with this project and publicly thank him for inviting me to join him. I'd also like to thank our agent, Margot Maley Hutchinson for her coaching and good humor. In addition, I'm grateful to our editor Matthew Lore for his faith in this project, and his assistant, Courtney Napoles, who demonstrates unwavering kindness, hard work, and almost instant availability. I much appreciate those folks in the case studies and the professionals who help band patients—all of whom took the time and energy to allow me to pester them for interviews. And finally, I'd like to thank my spouse, Mark, for his support and faith in me throughout my band journey.

Linda Rohrbough
April 2007
www.LindaRohrbough.com

Index